RELAX AND FEEL GOOD

RELAX AND FEEL GOOD

Make Relaxation Your Key to Energy and Well Being

Hilary Peters

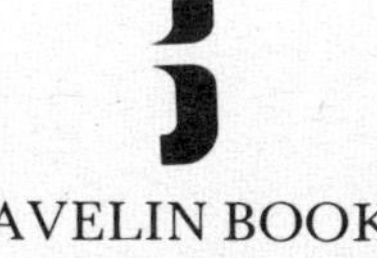

JAVELIN BOOKS
POOLE · NEW YORK · SYDNEY

First published in the UK 1986 by Javelin Books,
Link House, West Street, Poole, Dorset BH15 1LL

Distributed in the United States by
Sterling Publishing Co., Inc.,
2 Park Avenue, New York, NY 10016

Distributed in Australia by
Capricorn Link (Australia) Pty Ltd,
PO Box 665, Lane Cove, NSW 2066

ISBN 0 7137 1780 7

British Library Cataloguing in Publication Data

Peters, Hilary
Relax and feel good : make relaxation your key
to energy and well being.
1. Relaxation
I. Title
613.7'9 RA785

Typeset by Word Perfect 99 Ltd, Bournemouth, Dorset.

Printed in Great Britain by Guernsey Press Ltd

To Rose Hacker
who first taught me to relax

CONTENTS

Introduction 9
1 What Stops You Letting Go? 14
2 Exercise 21
3 Relaxation: the 30-Day Plan 36
4 Relaxing for Particular Complaints 75
5 Relaxing in Particular Circumstances 103
Appendices 123
Bibliography 125
Index 126

INTRODUCTION

The systematic teaching of relaxation for therapy started with Jacobson in World War I. Anyone who teaches tightening the muscles and letting them go is building on his foundations.

Laura Mitchell added a slight variation in her 'physiological method' when she recommended stretching the groups of muscles opposite to the ones held in tension, in order to induce relaxation. Most relaxation teachers combine these two methods and any others that work for their particular pupils. I am no exception.

The drawback to all books on relaxation is that reading about and doing are two different activities. The main point of reading this book is to follow the 30-day plan in Chapter 3. The reading is only intended as a way in to the doing. You may find a better way in (like getting someone to read the instructions to you or reading them into a cassette-recorder).

If you do use a cassette-player in learning to relax, it is worth investing in one that turns itself off.

I teach relaxation. That, in itself, takes some explaining. There are three main groups of eyebrow-raisers when I say that, and I tend to make the wrong explanation to the wrong group.

Group 1 is people to whom relaxation means watching television or going on holiday. To them, it is the last activity, in a world of spoon feeding, which needs to be taught.

Group 2 is members of the medical hierarchy, who vary from

those who think relaxation is a code word for some fraudulent religion, through those who recommend it when all else fails, to those who practise it themselves but it is hypnosis.
Group 3 is other alternative therapists. We don't always know as much about each other as we might.

So I'd like to start by defining what I do and how I came to do it.

I might as well admit that I came to relaxation through religion. I read theology as a student, but not much of it was about religion. I did yoga for many years. Not much of that was about religion either. Both were valuable and fun, but both were about achievement: one intellectual, the other physical. Religion is about letting go, and that means letting go of achievement too.

Religion, for me, is anything that breaks down the barrier between me and the rest of the world. Obviously different things do that for different people. But a common ingredient of them all is relaxing: actually letting go of the physical muscles. When you are tense, you are shut off in your personal prison. When you are relaxed, you are part of the whole. It is your decision how much you want to be an individual and how much a part of the whole. Most religious systems offer a way of surrendering individuality which goes much further than people bargain for, but the actual method of relaxing is a skill anyone can learn.

Since physical relaxation is a skill, you can learn it independently of the system it supports. It has never played much part in Western Christianity. So it seems outlandish to people brought up in the Western tradition. To some, that is an advantage: it is exotic, unchristian. To others, that is a cause for suspicion. Both are equally misguided. Relaxation is *only* a basic physical skill.

Yoga, as it is taught in this country, tends to appeal to an élite. It works, but it is pretty demanding in time, in fitness, in concentration. Yoga aims to transform you, so there's not much point in taking it up if you don't want to be transformed. If you do, it takes you still further away from the problems of the rest of the world – you could say that is the fault of the rest of the world. (If you want to learn about yoga, read Iyengar's *Light on Yoga*. To learn yoga, go to a class. Classes are run in most areas. *Yoga: 28-Day Exercise Plan* by Richard Hittleman is a good introduction.)

But I was looking for something everyone can do. Relaxation appealed to me as the basic common denominator. Everyone does it naturally to some extent. So why should they want to learn it? Usually because they have been told to do so by a doctor. This is what happened to Amber Lloyd's husband after he had had a heart attack. She formed *Relaxation for Living* in the UK in reply to this challenge. *R for L* trains relaxation teachers. So we all teach roughly the same material, bringing very different approaches to it. We all give a 6- to 8-week course of weekly classes to small groups. Many of our pupils are referred to us by doctors and psychiatrists. Some just want to learn.

The classes consist of some theory about stress and practice in recognising it in ourselves and others, some physiological explanation of how stress affects the body and discussion of stress related diseases, some loosening exercises for releasing tension, a little massage, and a weekly talk-down towards deep relaxation. This book is no substitute for a course of relaxation classes. It is more like an introduction.

Tightening and letting go is the rhythm of life. Tightening and not letting go causes stress problems.

When do we fail to let go?

We start early.

Fear of failure, or, where failure is pre-supposed, despair, are instilled into our children.

Later in life, they come out as worry, panic attacks, insomnia, depression, migraine, hypertension, phobias, a perpetual tightening in the stomach and guts that leads to stomach ulcers and colitis, a tightening in the neck and shoulders that leads to fibrositis, frozen shoulder, headaches, that total tightening up in self-defence that becomes arthritis.

For these and many more tension-related ailments there is a formula which must, at least, alleviate. Don't aim, at this stage, for a cure. Aim for an improvement.

1 Recognise your tension.
2 Increase it.
3 Let it go.
4 Keep on letting go.

I will elaborate this in Chapter 4, applying it to particular problems.

But first, a few warnings:

1 *Relaxation works but you won't get instant results.* A month of patient work may produce the same result as one pill. So why not take the pill? Because it has side-effects.

2 *Relaxation is ONLY not doing. That's all it is.* You have to keep on at relaxation, but it is no good working too hard or too dutifully at it. You cannot relax by trying. People who stick very dutifully to this or any other formula and put a lot of effort into getting it right, are less likely to reach relaxation than those who take it less seriously. Be on the look-out all the time for relaxation taking over and teaching you. *Don't try, but persevere.* You'll never relax by making an effort.

3 *Relaxation is cumulative.* You may not feel it at first, but in fact every suggestion your brain makes to your muscles produces some result. It may not be the result you want. Perhaps you have stronger reasons for not wanting to relax than for wanting to relax? (For being ill than for being well?) You will learn more about yourself, inevitably, as you learn to relax. Perhaps you don't want to know yourself better?

4 *When you have got used to the feel of relaxation (which is very pleasant), there will be times when you can't feel it any more.* These may be the

times when you most need it, e.g. coming round from an anaesthetic. Don't let this worry you. The whole point of an anaesthetic is to destroy feeling. Just keep relaxing. The feeling will come back. (It may take as long as a week.)

5 *There will be times when relaxing brings out more pain.* Tensions will come to the surface as you relax – maybe tensions you didn't know you had. You may get worse before you get better. This applies to mental pain too. You have built up your tensions for good reasons – to guard yourself from things you can't face. Before you destroy your armour, be sure you can do without it.

6 *Instead of releasing tension, it's possible to shift it around.* Pain in the neck can become pain in the back. Compulsive smoking, cured, can surface again as compulsive eating. The structure of your tensions is complicated. Be sure you want to learn to relax before you start.

1

WHAT STOPS YOU LETTING GO?

Exercise and relaxation are two halves of the same activity; you can't have one without the other.

The heart rests for as long as it pumps (slightly longer).

The lungs expand and contract.

You spend hours awake and hours asleep.

This sort of balance goes all through life, whether we want it to or not.

Trouble starts when we upset the balance.

There are three basic ways of upsetting the balance.

1 *Too much exercise.* You can do too much, like the athlete who is too exhausted to sleep. In this case, you need to recognise the moment when your performance falls off, however much energy you spend. You must learn to relax before that moment arrives in order to improve your performance.

2 *Too much relaxation.* You can do too little, like the depressive who lacks the will to get out of bed in the morning. Again, it is important to see this moment coming and stimulate yourself with small rewards in order to get going.

3 *Holding up the process.* You can block the flow of energy at any point along the line.

This book is mostly about blocking the flow of energy – where and how and why we create blocks for ourselves and what we can do to dissolve them.

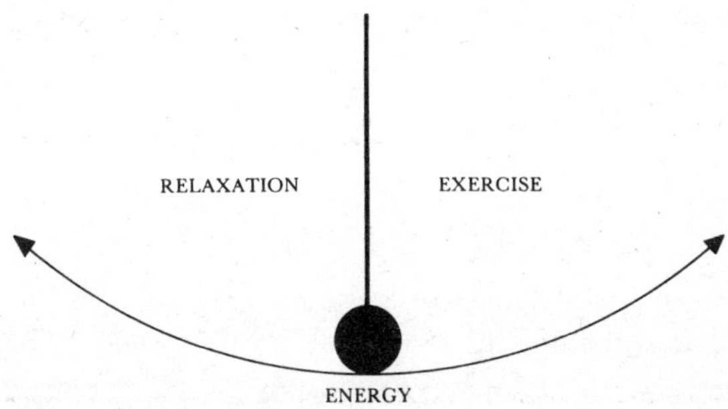

The more you relax, the more you are tapping a fund of energy.
The more of this energy you spend in exercise, the more deeply you are able to relax.
If you stop the flow at any point, you block the energy.

We block the natural flow of exercise and relaxation by holding on to emotions. Consider what happens when you have a shock:

1 The message is received in the brain (like pressing an alarm button).
2 The hypothalamus (or alarm button) instantly prepares the body for action by passing the message to the pituitary gland.
3 The pituitary co-ordinates all the other glands and so hormones are produced all over the body.

Simultaneously:

The heart rate increases.
The breathing speeds up.
The stomach pumps acid into the system.
The liver releases sugar into the bloodstream.
The brain becomes more active.
The adrenal glands work overtime.
The muscles tense.
The digestion slows down.
The reproductive system stops working.
The saliva dries up.
The skin sweats.
The pupils dilate.

The hair stands on end.

The anti-inflammatory system stops working.

The blood becomes ready to clot.

The excretory system closes down.

The body is then ready to fight, to run away or to preserve itself if wounded.

As long as you *do* fight or run away, *physically*, the hormones produced will fulfil their normal function. Your life will be preserved and the shock to the system will do you no harm. In fact, such shocks are necessary to the normal functioning of the body.

It is when you can't fight or run away, or when you fall into the habit of having this reaction in a situation where it is no longer appropriate, that you lay the foundations of stress diseases.

We seldom, if ever, have the chance to fight or run away, yet we have shocks (annoyances, disappointments, anxieties) many times a day. So, what do we do instead? *We tighten the muscles*. Imagine that you have just had a shock and check what you do. The possibilities seem endless. You might:

Hold your breath.

Pull in your stomach muscles.

Clench your fists.

Tighten your buttock muscles.

Raise your shoulders.

Put pressure on your hip joints, knee joints or ankle joints.

Clench your teeth.

Screw up your eyes.

Arch your neck or your back.

Curl your toes.

Push your elbows into your ribs.

Hold your thighs together.

These are some of the more common responses. Find out what *you* do. It doesn't have to be just one thing. When you have identified your habitual reaction, you will probably find that it centres either around the top of the spine (shoulders, neck, jaw, eyes, face, arms and hands) or the base of the spine (buttock muscles, stomach muscles, hip joints, lower back, legs and feet).

Your responses may fall into both categories but, if they fall very definitely into one or the other, you may be able to find out more about *why* you tighten by studying *where* you tighten.

1 *Tightening at the top of the spine* (leading to headaches, frozen shoulder, fibrositis, laryngitis, pain in elbow and finger joints among other things) is a way of *repressing anger*.

2 *Tightening at the base of the spine* (leading to stomach and bowel upsets, ulcers, colitis, pain in the hip joints, knees, ankles, feet and lumbago) is a way of *repressing fear*.

This is not hard and fast. Anger and fear are so mixed together anyway that it may not be worth the bother of unravelling them. However, this is a rough guide to finding out what you do and why.

What is your weak spot? You probably have a place where you tighten habitually, whatever the shock. If you have, feel it now and imagine the sort of situation in which you tighten there. Try to feel what it is that you are holding on to. I don't mean remember back to the first time you tightened there. That would be impossible and, even if you could recall the original cause, unprofitable. It is what you are doing *now* that is relevant; the muscles you are using *now*; the feelings you are repressing *now*. Do you:

Frown . . . to scare the enemy?
Stare . . . to reduce the power that is hostile to you?
Stick your jaw forward . . . in stubborn refusal?
Clench your teeth . . . to bite back your pain?
Clamp your tongue to the roof of your mouth . . . in apprehension?
Tighten your throat . . . to prevent yourself vomiting?
Arch your neck . . . to take cover?

Jut your head forward . . . from under your shell?
Raise your shoulders . . . to ward off attack?
Roll your shoulders forward . . . to bear the load?
Push your elbows into your ribs . . . to hold yourself together?
Tighten your forearms, wrists, hands . . . to hit out?
Hold your breath . . . to gain control?
Hold your stomach muscles in . . . to withstand attack?
Arch your back . . . to protect your genitals?
Tighten your buttock muscles . . . to hold your guts steady?
Contract your thigh muscles and groin . . . to say no to sexual suggestion?
Pull your knees back . . . in anger?
Tighten your calf muscles . . . to run away?
Hold your feet up . . . in unease?
Screw up your toes . . . in embarrassment?

To take one example, this is what I do, although I react in most of the other ways as well.

At the first intimation of anything I suspect may prove unbearable, *I tighten the tendons at the side of my neck.* This tightens the whole top of my spine, so that I grind my head downwards, sticking my neck out.

This feels like some sort of armour against anything which I don't want to see or hear. I'm a stiff-necked person, although actually I never get a stiff neck. The mental attitude this gesture embodies is: *No. I can't bear it and I won't.* A lot of other tightenings follow from this basic one; the jaw, tongue, face, eyes all tighten up automatically (tension headaches); the shoulders rise and come forwards and the muscles tighten all the way down the arms (I often get pins and needles in the fingers); the tension spreads down the spine, so I clench my hip joints and tighten all the way down the legs as well.

So, one basic response of avoidance affects the whole body. What can I do about it?

1 *Recognise it*

Generally, I don't until I have a headache. It is a very slight movement, invisible to most observers. (Anyone can feel it easily by putting their fingers on the sides of my neck.) But, if I stop to feel, it is quite easily recognised from the inside.

So, I need to know I'm doing it and to recognise what I'm blocking off. Is what I'm avoiding really unbearable? It may be something quite trivial. If it *is* unbearable, perhaps I should do something about it? Am I the *only* person who finds it unbearable? If so, do I need to change myself rather than the world?

What is unbearable about it? I might try to find a way of expressing this emotion instead of burying it in the neck. I might feel it starting, taking hold, dying down. I probably don't do this because I fear it never will die down. I'd rather it festered in the neck than took over the whole of my consciousness.

2 *Loosen the physical block*

(a) With fingers pressing the back of my neck, roll my head gently until I get a click or two.
(b) Roll my head to each extreme position, not forcing.
(c) Drop my head sideways towards each shoulder in turn.
(d) Massage my own neck and tops of shoulders.
(e) Waggle my jaw.
(f) Roll my shoulders backwards.
(g) Roll my eyes.

These, done once, will probably make the problem worse but loosening exercises, done regularly, do make for greater mobility. If everything is mobile, it is much more difficult to get stuck.

So, once I've got things moving, I need to relax in order to keep them on the move.

3 *Learn deep relaxation*

I have. It works for me, which is my qualification for writing this book.

It is cumulative, so don't expect miracles the first day, but, if you follow the 30-day plan in Chapter 3 of this book and feel no different at the end, you should check several things:

(a) *What drugs you are on*

Tranquillisers, anti-depressants, pain-killers, anaesthetics will take over your natural powers of relaxation so that, in the early stages of learning relaxation, you may not feel much. This is not an excuse for giving up. In time, you may be able to replace your drugs with relaxation, but be patient. If you are coming off drugs, always consult a doctor.

(b) *Whether you'd rather be ill than well*

Pain in the neck is uncomfortable, headaches incapacitating, blood clots in the brain a reminder of the end, but they may all be preferable to the mental pain I am running away from.

(c) *Whether you try too hard*

Trying to relax is a contradiction. If you follow orders very dutifully, fix your mind on getting it right, put a lot of effort into it and are ambitious to excel, you are likely to get less benefit out of it than someone who doesn't try, but perseveres. There is a subtle shift of the attention from giving orders with the mind to receiving impressions with the mind. It is this passive, but alert, state that is conducive to relaxation.

If you don't know what I'm talking about, try trying not to try.

(d) *Whether you are in the stage of tensions coming out*

Many people feel worse when they first start to relax. Getting through life is mainly a matter of balancing one tension against another. If you have evolved some sort of balance that works for you, however painfully, you may feel letting go of your tensions is uncomfortable, or worse. This stage will pass if you persevere.

(e) *Whether you are just moving tensions around*

It is easy to concentrate so hard on letting go in one part of the body that you tighten up somewhere else. If you do this, you may lose the pain that drove you to relaxation, but develop something else. It is necessary to check constantly. Relaxation should make you more aware, not less.

2

EXERCISE

Exercise should be a pleasure in its own right, not a duty performed with a specific aim. Whatever you do, apart from deep relaxation, you are exercising some muscles. The object of the exercises in this book is to do whatever you do already with greater awareness and less restraint.

So, if exercise is whatever you do anyway, what are you doing now? What muscles are you using? What muscles are you stopping yourself from using?

If you can make your everyday life your gymnasium, you will be tackling the problem where it is, which is not at all the same thing as doing nothing about it.

Start with the principle of letting go *into* whatever you are doing instead of tightening up *against* it.

Warning: It is hard enough to teach exercises to someone who is standing beside you. To start with, these are not exercises in the sense of physical jerks. They are just movements to release tension. One test of 'getting it right' is whether you feel looser in joints and muscles. If you are tenser, stop doing them and go to a class. At best this chapter is a way in. Do not take it as the last word on exercises.

Before you start doing specific exercises, think of your body as a puppet on a string. The pull of gravity will then extend, instead of contracting, all your joints. Feel the pull upwards through the spine. Feel yourself moving in this extended way.

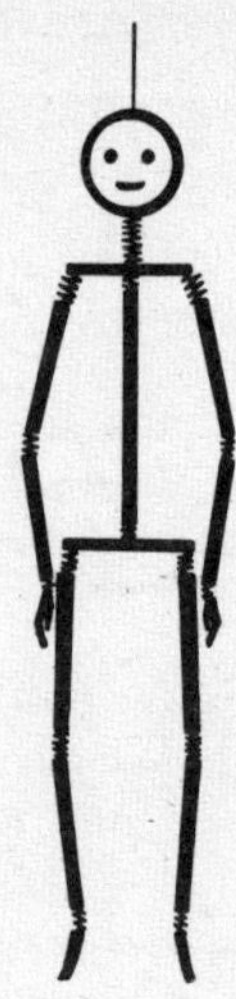

1 RISING

Notice your position in bed when you wake. If you sleep with your arms over your head (warding off the world?), you will have a lot of tension in the shoulders and neck. Do you wake with pins and needles in your fingers? This comes from tension at the back of the neck. If you sleep with your teeth held together, or grind them in your sleep, your jaw is probably tense all the time. Notice if your tongue is on the roof of your mouth when you wake. It is a sign of tension.

EXERCISES

1 Lie on your back and stretch. Start gradually with your extremities.

Have a rest between each stretch but keep going until you have stretched the whole spine.

Yawn too, but gently at first.

If you can roll from side to side as you yawn, this also loosens the spine.

Don't get up until you have done this. Give yourself a couple of minutes of stretching, yawning and rolling.

Notice how you get up, especially if you are stiff at the base of the spine. It is important not to sit bolt upright from lying flat on your back. Always roll over on your side and sit up gently.

2 STANDING

EXERCISES

1 Stand as you usually stand.
Notice exactly what you do.
Is your weight on one leg?
Are your feet turned out?
Are you bracing your knees?
Are you arching your back?
Are you pushing your pelvis forwards?
Are you raising your shoulders?

2 Now stand, in turn, in four extreme positions:
(a) On your right leg with your left foot just resting on the floor. Your left knee will be bent and your right hip will be sticking out.

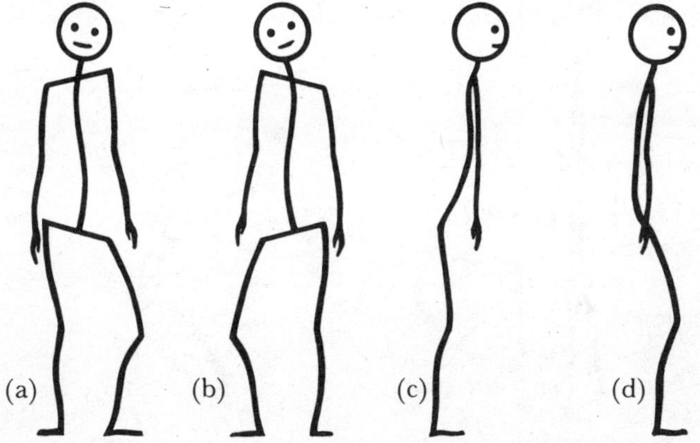

(b) On your left leg, with your left hip sticking out and your right leg bent.
(c) On both legs, arching your back, sticking out your bottom and tightening both knees.
(d) On both legs, sticking your pelvis forwards, tucking your bottom under and bending your knees slightly.

3 The standing position that is least strain lies between the four extremes above.
Have your feet slightly apart and parallel.
Feel the weight equally distributed between both feet.
Let your pelvis drop – don't hold it in any particular position.
Allow the spine to extend upwards.
Think upwards.
Imagine a string through the crown of your head. Whatever movement you make, the head leads.

Notice your standing position. Are you arching your back or pushing your pelvis forwards? If so, let go in the muscles at the

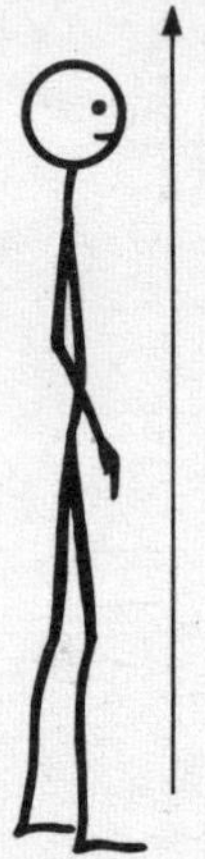

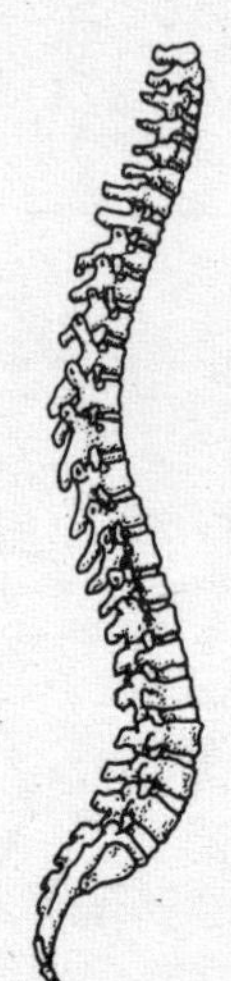

back of the waist. Check that the weight is equally on both legs. Find the standing position which is most comfortable for you.

3 WALKING

Walking should exercise every part of the body without inducing undue tension. But it depends how you walk. In any activity, you can use a maximum or a minimum number of muscles. The right number is just enough to get the job done efficiently.

Again, think of leading with the head. Don't *do* anything but direct your energy upwards.

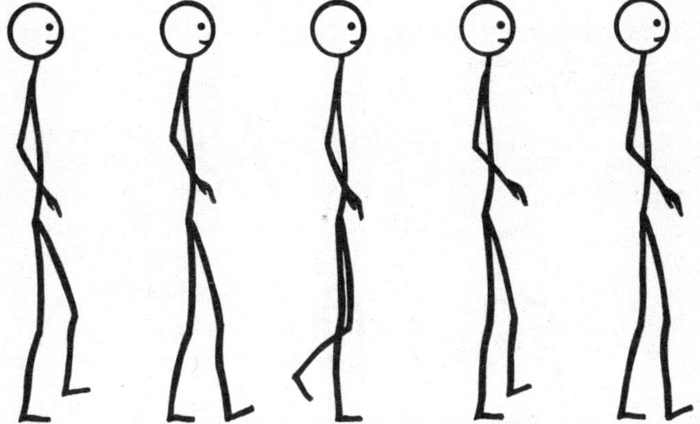

EXERCISES

1. Slow down your walk until you can feel every movement.
   Put one foot down. Feel exactly how it touches the ground, how you put your weight onto it and how you transfer the weight.
   Then, lift the other foot. Feel all the muscles which you use to do this.
   Feel exactly what happens when you transfer the weight.
   Where do you tighten?

Are your feet gripping the floor?
Are your ankles clenched?
Are you tightening the thigh or buttock muscles?
Do you:

Arch your back?
Hold your stomach in?
Raise your shoulders?
Clench your hands?
Stick your head forwards?
Grit your teeth?
Frown?
Stare?

Keep walking and watching.

To loosen the ankles:

2 Stand on one leg and roll the other foot from the ankle joint.
Both ways.
Do the other foot.

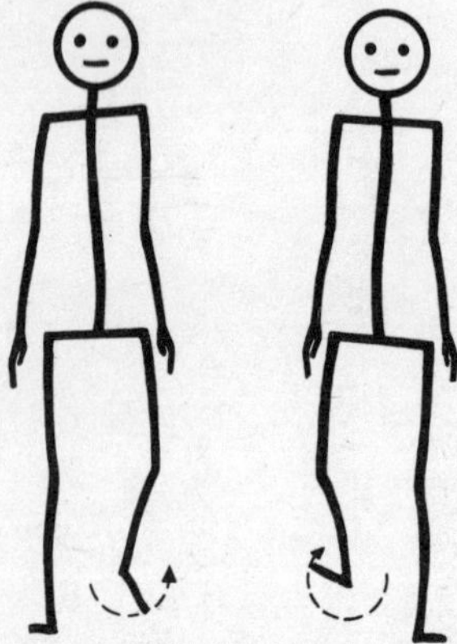

3 Hold the leg at the calf and let the foot go floppy.
Give it a good shake.
Shake the other foot.

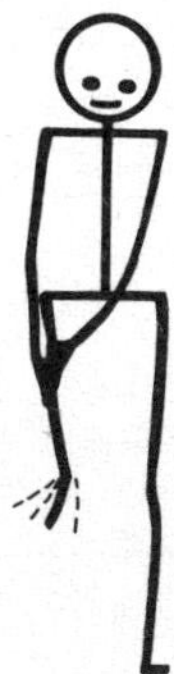

Cracks are releasing tension. Don't worry about them. But if you give yourself cramp, which is a guide to how tense you are, bend the foot upwards from the ankle. Massage the instep and sole of the foot. Foot massage, anyway, is an aid to relaxation.

To loosen the calf muscles:

4 Stand with the feet hip-width apart and parallel.
Rise onto your toes.
Put your heels down.
Bend your knees.

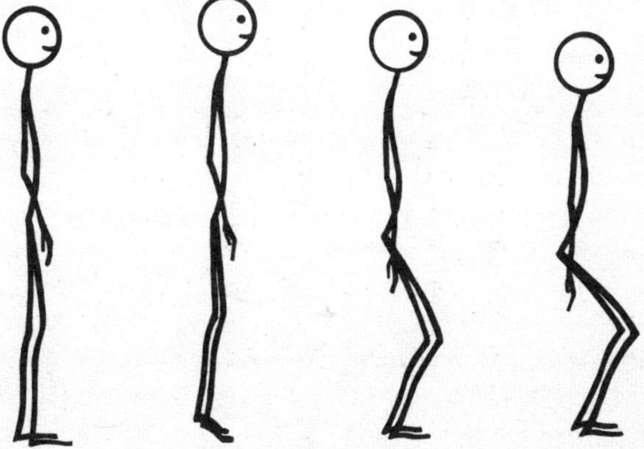

Go down as far as you can without taking your heels off the ground.
Repeat ten times.

5 Shake your legs one at a time.

To loosen the knees:

6 Stand with your knees together and parallel.
Put your hands on your knees and do a circular movement from the knee joints, first one way, then the other.

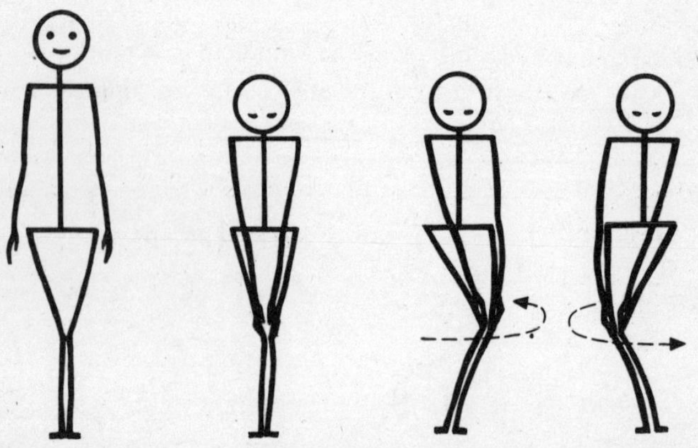

When you are walking, do you enjoy it? If you don't, why not? Is it something you can alter?
Get into the habit of feeling what's happening to your body, where you're tightening, why.
Walking can create tension or it can ease it. Notice if you use your jaw, your shoulders or your fingers as you walk. Notice your breathing. Be aware of what's happening in your mind as well.

If you walk a couple of miles a day, you probably won't find relaxing so difficult.

4 SITTING AT A DESK

Sitting at a desk is many people's commonest activity, so it's worth paying some attention to how you get there and what you sit on, before getting down to the actual activity.

In sitting down, it is usual to place a lot of unnecessary strain on the spine. (For a full description of how to sit down, see Wilfred Barlow's *The Alexander Principle*.) Give yourself a chance, both in getting there, and when you're there, to keep the spine reasonably straight. Also see that your chair is the right height, especially if you're typing. It should be high enough to type without raising your shoulders. Once you're there, sit with your weight equally on both buttocks, your legs uncrossed and your feet flat on the floor.

EXERCISES

The main problems among desk-workers occur in the shoulders and neck. The following exercises should help to relax the muscles in the shoulders.

1 Shrug one shoulder.
Then the other.
Then both.

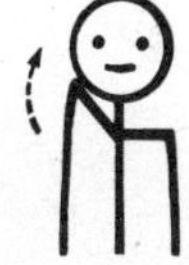
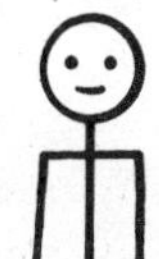
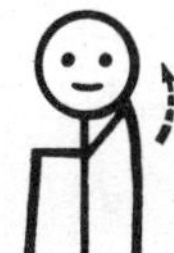
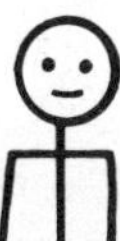
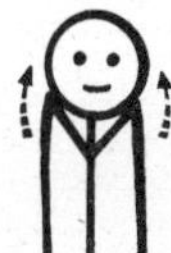
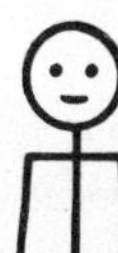

2 Rotate one shoulder.
Lift it.
Take it back.
Drop it.
Bring it forward.
Then the other.
Then both.

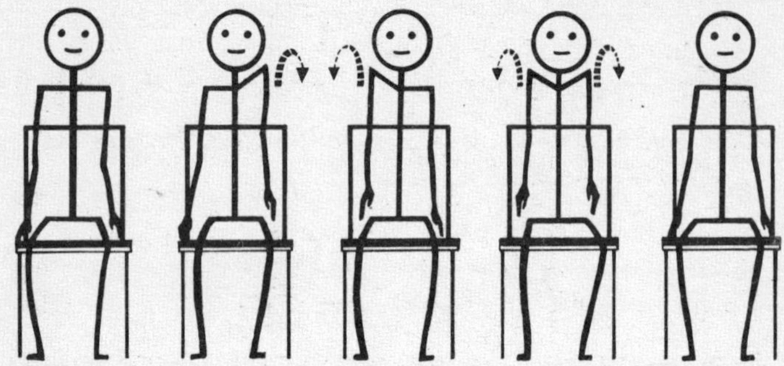

3 Hold your arms roughly halfway between shoulder height and vertical, out to the sides.
Moving from your shoulder joints, describe a circle with your hands.

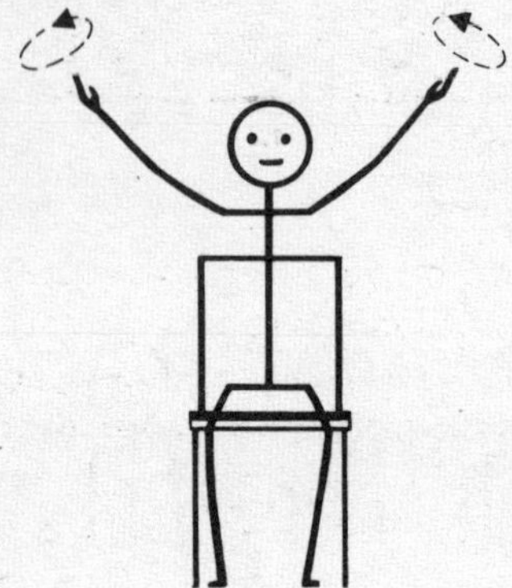

You can do all these exercises quite a lot.

For the neck:

4 Drop your head forward. Roll it to one side. Then round to the back. Then to the other side. Do this very gently at first. Come back if there is pain. If you don't like it, move your head in a much smaller circle.

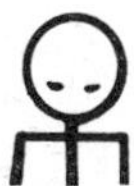 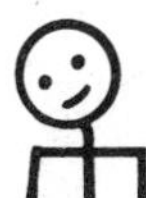  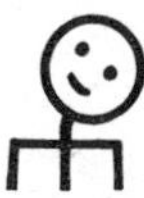

5 Drop your head towards your right shoulder. Then the left. Don't raise your shoulder.

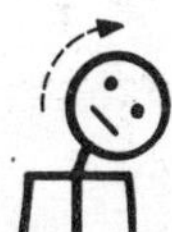 

6 With your elbow on the desk, with your chin cupped in your left hand. Use your right hand, pull your head gently round to the left. Pause. Change hands and repeat to the right.

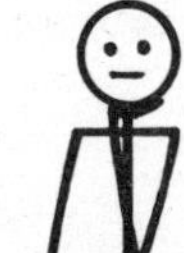 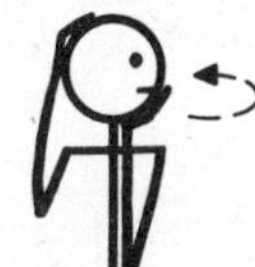 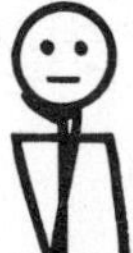 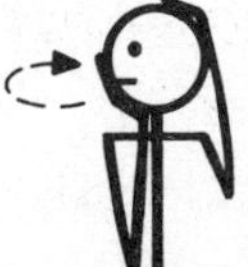

With all neck exercises, be gentle.

For the whole spine:

7 Sit straight, with both feet flat on the floor. Bend over to the right as if you had something heavy in the left hand. Then bend to the left. All movement is in the spine.
Do this several times, feel the arms and spine lengthening.

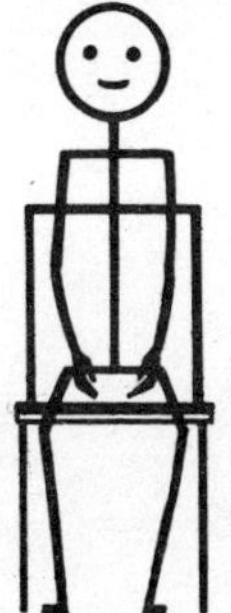 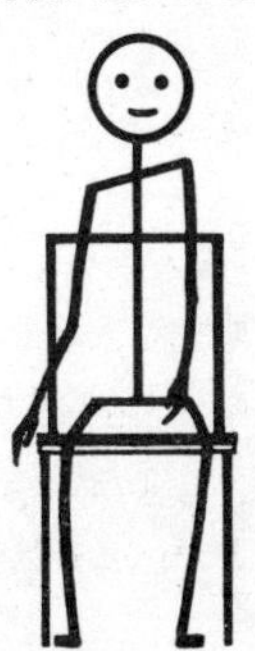 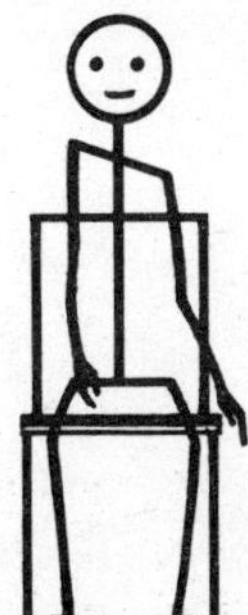

5 HOUSEWORK

Housework can be a useful exercise or a source of suffering, particularly in the back (and mind) Anything that involves stooping and bending forward is more easily done by bending the knees than by moving from the waist.

If you do a lot of lifting, remember to use the leg muscles rather than the back muscles.

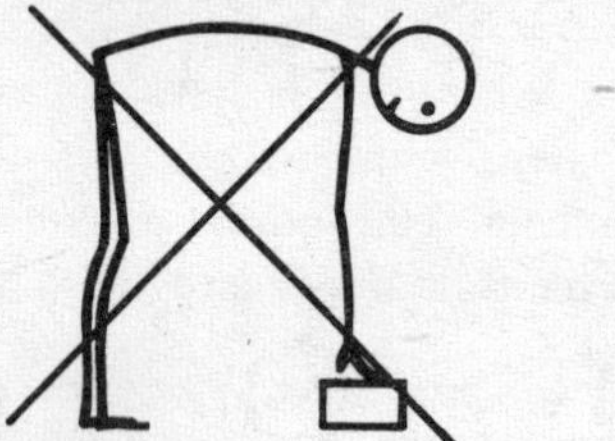

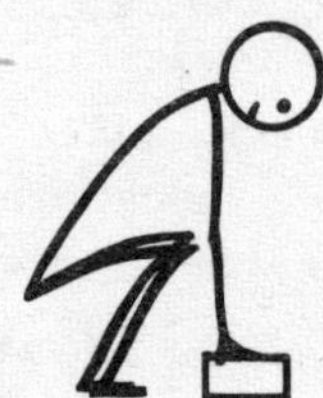

EXERCISES

1 To uncurl the spine, stand with the feet hip-width apart and hands on hips.
  Bend backwards from the hips.
  Do this several times but do not stay in the extreme position.

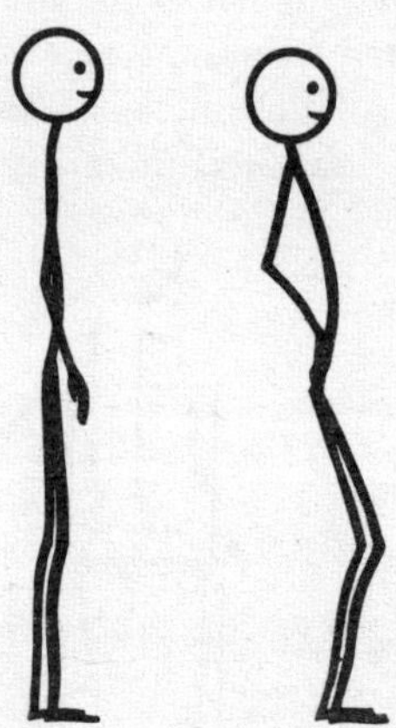

2 Shake your arms and hands like an Olympic swimmer preparing for a race.

If hating your work is a problem, try concentrating on the mechanical details of doing it rather than on the end product, e.g. I am now picking up a knife in my right hand and a potato in my left. What muscles am I using? This works with deep relaxation as well. You don't try to bring about an imagined change. You focus on specific groups of muscles.

6 SITTING IN AN ARMCHAIR

Reading and watching television, usually classified as relaxation, can be one of our most stressful occupations. Notice how you sit. Is your spine twisted? Are you slumped on your tail-bone? Is the object of your attention below eye-level? Are you using hand, arm or jaw muscles?

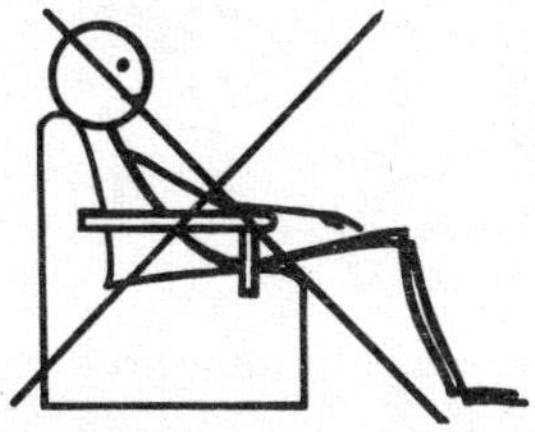

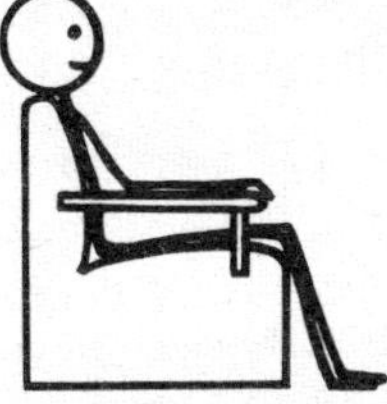

An easy chair should be one in which you can be at ease, with your spine straight (it does not have to be upright), your head supported and your shoulders down. If you read a lot, a book-rest could help. There is no reason why your eye-muscles and brain should not be the only active parts of you.

EXERCISES

The following exercises will help you to relax your eyes:

1 Sitting at ease, hold up one finger about 18 inches (45 centimetres) in front of you, or wherever you can focus on it comfortably.

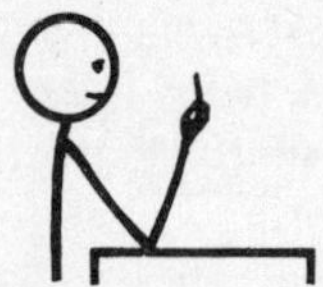

Stare at it.
Blink.
Widen your gaze and look past your finger.
Blink.
Repeat several times.

2 Roll your eyes.
Look up.
Look to your right.
Look down.
Look to your left.
Blink.

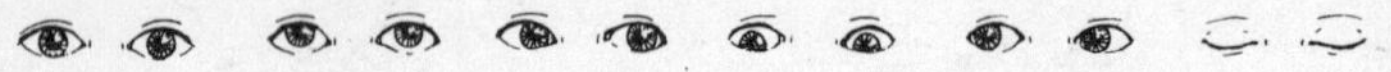

Repeat in the opposite direction.

3 Place the heels of your hands gently in your eye-sockets.
Hold them there, seeing nothing.
Relax in this position with your elbows supported.
(This is Bates' 'palming' and it takes time to get anything out of it, especially for people with good eyesight. It is worth persevering with it until you find it working.)

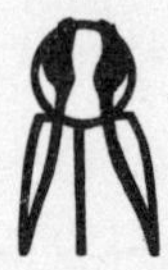

For the whole body:

4 Before settling into a sitting position, stretch the whole body.
Extend the back of the neck, legs, arms and spine.
Settle with the spine as straight as possible.
Do this once more before getting up.

3

RELAXATION: THE 30-DAY PLAN

Relaxation, as well as exercise, is something you do naturally. It is a question of re-learning an old skill rather than inventing something new.

When I tell people I teach relaxation, these are the two commonest comments:

'I don't need to relax. I need to get going.'

'I can relax my body all right. It's my mind.'

Relaxation is not the same as playing squash or going on holiday or watching television. Indeed, it is often the opposite. It is the state of the body and mind when no muscles are being used. When you reach this state, you become aware of a fund of energy.

This state when no muscles are being used is not natural in our society. We don't reach it in sleep, or in the sports and hobbies we call relaxation. So it is hard to convey the feel of relaxation to people who have not known it for themselves.

The way to get there is by a lot of physical *doing*, although relaxation itself is essentially *not doing. Not doing* is not at all that state of blank inertia brought on by a block. That is more a kind of anti-doing.

To reach relaxation, you *do* and then *stop doing* a set of basic physical activities.

But relaxation is not the doing, nor the stopping doing. It is what happens when you stop doing. It may take time to feel this.

How long?

It varies from person to person. I should practise for at least 5 minutes twice a day at first.

You may reach a stage when you can feel your muscles relaxing, but not your mind. This is just a stage. Given time, the one will spill over into the other. For many people, the muscles of speech and vision act as the bridge.

N.B. This is not designed to be read as literature. There is no point at all in reading this section unless you mean to *do* it.

DAY ONE THE HANDS

SITTING

1 Clench your fists . . . as much as you can. Keep clenching and notice where else you tighten.
2 Let go.
3 Put your hands on something, finger tips down. Feel. Shut your eyes and register the feeling of letting go in all your finger joints. Can you feel anywhere else letting go? Notice what's happening to your breathing. If you can't feel much, tighten once more, briefly. Then give yourself time to concentrate on the feeling of letting go in the whole of both hands. Can you let go any more?

LYING

Lie flat on your back. If that is uncomfortable, prop yourself on cushions, but get as near to lying as you can:

1 Induce the minimum tension instead of the maximum in your fingers. Tighten just enough to feel something in each finger joint. Check that you are not holding your breath and notice what other parts of your body tighten in sympathy.
2 Let go.

3 Put your hands down beside you, palms down. Feel. Feel first what's happening in the finger joints. Make sure you're letting go everything you tightened. Is it possible to let go any more?

4 Check quickly through your body to see that you are not tightening:
   Wrists
   Elbows
   Shoulders
   Neck
   Jaw
   Tongue
   Eyes
   Facial muscles
   Spine
   Front of the body
   Stomach
   Buttocks
   Thighs
   Knees
   Calves
   Ankles
   Feet

5 Take your attention to your breathing. Don't alter it, but notice whether or not your whole body is letting go on the out-breath.

N.B. Don't force anything. Just watch it happening and be honest with yourself if it isn't happening. You are learning to observe the body rather than imposing orders on it. The orders (and there are plenty at the beginning) are only a stage. When you feel the relaxation working for yourself, you can give up the orders, or invent your own.

DAY TWO THE WRISTS

SITTING

1 Bend both wrists so that your hands are going downwards towards the forearms. Do what you like with your hands so as to feel most tension in the wrists.
2 Let go.
3 Put your finger tips on something. Have your forearms supported too so that you can feel the letting go in your wrists.

LYING

With the forearms parallel to your body, elbows wide:

1 Bend your wrists up so that your finger tips are just off the ground.
2 Let go.
3 Let the whole of both arms flop as much as you can and feel what is happening in your wrist joints.

N.B. Feeling is not something you can do from the outside like putting your hand on a muscle to feel it letting go. You are learning to feel from the inside. The muscles are sending back messages to the brain. All the brain has to do is receive them.

DAY THREE THE ELBOWS

SITTING

1 Push your elbows into your sides. Tighten anything else that follows on from that. Concentrate on squeezing your ribs with your elbows so that you are holding yourself together. Notice your breathing without altering it deliberately.

2 Let go.
3 Feel. Do this as many times as you need to feel what is happening, but spend at least twice as long on the letting go as on the tensing.

LYING

1 Minimum tension in the elbows, muscles between the ribs, and anywhere else?
2 Let go.
3 Feel.

For all these exercises exact timing is not important but, as a rough guide:
Let go for twice as long as you tighten.
Don't practise at first for much longer than 5 minutes at a time but do at least 5 minutes twice a day.

N.B. Daily practice is really necessary.

DAY FOUR THE SHOULDERS

SITTING

Begin to pay some attention to your sitting posture. Sit in an easy chair with a high back. You need to be able to rest your head against something at first. Don't cross your legs; have your feet flat on the floor, your weight equally on both buttocks and your back supported. If the chair has arms, make sure that when your hands are on them, your shoulders are down. If this is not possible, put your hands in your lap.

1 Pull your shoulders up around your ears. Do anything else that you usually do to express tension in the shoulders, e.g. clench your fists if you need to. Be aware of other parts that tighten up in sympathy.

2 Let go.
3 Feel the letting go. When you think you've felt all you can, let go a bit more through the shoulder joints.

LYING

1 Induce the least possible tension in your shoulders. Be aware of what's happening down your arms, up your neck and down your spine.
2 Let go.
3 Feel. Each time you breathe out, feel what's happening in the shoulder joints. Don't alter your breathing. Just notice.

N.B. Most of us hold our shoulders permanently up a little. When you notice this, don't start holding them down. Relaxing is simply *not doing*. It isn't doing something different.

DAY FIVE RECAPITULATION DAY

SITTING IN AN EASY CHAIR

Be comfortable. Support your head. Make sure your spine is not twisted and that you are not holding yourself together with your hands.

1 Clench your fists.
2 Let go.
3 Feel.
4 Tighten your wrists.
5 Let go.
6 Feel.
7 Tense your elbows.
8 Let go.
9 Feel. And keep on feeling and letting go.

10 Hunch your shoulders.
11 Let go.
12 Feel the letting go through the shoulder joints and right down both arms.

LYING

See that your weight is falling equally on each side of the body. Both heels, both buttocks, both shoulder blades and both hands should feel an equal pressure unless there is some physical reason why not. See that your head is reasonably straight to start with. Having straightened it out, you can let it drop to one side if it's really uncomfortable. Have the elbows wide from the body and the palms down. It's easier to feel like that at first. You can turn the hands over later if you want to.

If you have any pain at the base of the spine, put a cushion under your knees. If it's still painful, place a cushion under the arch of your back. Have your knees up, feet flat on the floor, or prop yourself up, depending on how bad it is. Do not attempt to relax into a pain at the base of the spine. Other pains, unless they are agony, are better relaxed into than run away from.

1 Clench your fists the least possible to feel it.
2 Let go.
3 Feel. Make sure you can feel what's happening in each finger and thumb joint and in the palms of your hands. Be especially aware of feeling as you breathe out.
4 Tighten your wrists minimally.
5 Let go.
6 Let your hands flop and notice if you're still using the wrist joints.
7 Induce minimal tension in your elbows.
8 Let go.
9 Tense a little through your shoulder joints.
10 Let go.

11 Feel through your shoulders.
12 Watch your breathing without altering it. Whether you want to or not, you take in energy on the in-breath and let go on the out-breath. Can you feel this happening?
13 When you've felt all you can (don't worry if it's nothing), let go a bit more in the fingers on the next out-breath. (If this sounds like nonsense, do it anyway.)
14 Next out-breath, feel what is happening in your wrists.
15 Next out-breath, the elbows.
16 Next out-breath, the shoulders. And concentrate on the shoulders for another two out-breaths.
17 Forget about the breathing but carry on feeling the letting go from shoulder joints to finger tips.
18 Go back to feeling the breathing. Feel the whole process.
19 The next three out-breaths, when you're ready, let go from the shoulders to the hands.

N.B. Letting go on the out-breath is not the same as a breathing exercise. You don't alter your normal breathing pattern in any way. You just coincide concentrating on the part you are letting go with a particular out-breath.

DAY SIX THE NECK

SITTING IN AN EASY CHAIR WITH A HIGH BACK

1 Tighten in your neck. This is most usually done by pushing the head out and then raising the chin (two movements) until all the pressure is concentrated in the bottom joint of the neck. You may normally do one or the other of these movements, or both. Do what is habitual for you.
2 Let go.
3 Drop your head onto the support so that you are using no

neck muscles at all. Give yourself time to feel all that's going on in the neck.

LYING

Check your position. Support your head with a pillow but make sure your shoulders are not on it too. The edge of the pillow should go through the middle of your neck.

1 Arch your neck slightly, just enough to feel tension. Although this is a very small movement, made sure you feel something and that you know what you are feeling.
2 Let go.
3 Feel what is happening in your neck. On each out-breath, concentrate on your neck. Feel the top joints of your spine. Feel the tendons at the side of your neck. Feel your throat loosening (if it is). If it isn't, swallow once, and then feel inside your throat as you breathe out.

N.B. Don't force yourself to feel what you think you ought to be feeling. Concentrate on what is actually happening.

DAY SEVEN THE JAW

SITTING IN AN UPRIGHT CHAIR

If this is your normal working position, sit as you usually do. Otherwise, have your legs uncrossed, your feet flat on the floor, your spine reasonably straight and your hands in your lap.

1 Tighten your jaw. Clench your teeth. Tighten everything that follows on. Notice the position of your tongue.
2 Let go.
3 Let your tongue rest on the lower jaw if it will. Feel yourself letting go through the hinges of your jaw.

LYING

1 Tighten your jaw and any facial muscles that seem to join in. Do this just enough to feel tension in your jaw.
2 Let go.
3 Let your jaw sag. Make sure your teeth are not still together even if your lips are. Begin to be aware of your breathing and of letting go through the hinges of the jaw on each out-breath.

N.B. Don't expect anything. Just feel.

DAY EIGHT THE TONGUE

SITTING IN AN UPRIGHT CHAIR

1 Squeeze your tongue against the roof of your mouth.
2 Let go.
3 Let your tongue drop onto your lower jaw and allow yourself to let go from the roots of your tongue. Feel the skin inside your mouth letting go.

LYING

1 Roll your tongue up, not too hard.
2 Let go.
3 Feel your tongue subsiding onto your lower jaw as you breathe out. If it doesn't, don't hold it down. Let it assume its natural position and then let go from the roots of the tongue as you breathe out.

N.B. Check in everyday life to see if your tongue is on the roof of your mouth. If it is, bring it gently down and watch what happens. Don't hold it down.

DAY NINE THE EYES

SITTING ON AN UPRIGHT CHAIR

1 Look straight ahead at some object about 2 feet (60 centimetres) away. Really stare at it. Focus your whole gaze on it. Then look beyond it and widen your gaze. Then blink and focus on the object again. Stare.
2 Close your eyes gently.
3 Feel your eye-muscles letting go.

LYING COMFORTABLY

1 Screw up your eyelids and all facial muscles that follow on.
2 Let go, letting your eyeballs fall back behind closed eyelids.
3 Feel what's happening to your eye-muscles and behind the eyes. Keep allowing yourself to let go between the eyes and behind the eyes as you breathe out.

N.B. If you go on seeing behind closed eyelids, don't try to stop yourself, but be aware of what you see. Watch what's happening without trying to interfere.

DAY TEN RECAPITULATION DAY

SITTING IN AN EASY CHAIR

With head supported, arms and hands supported, and legs uncrossed:

1 Tighten in your neck. Be sure you know your habitual way of tensing your neck, e.g. notice if you tighten the tendons at the sides of your neck. You may not necessarily move the joints at all. Notice what happens in the lungs.
2 Let go with your head supported.

3 Feel the weight of your head. Have you let go as much as you can in the top joints of your spine? . . . In your throat? In the sides of your neck? Feel the weight at the back of your neck.
4 Clench your teeth. Tighten inside the mouth. Tighten through the hinges of your jaw.
5 Let go.
6 Feel the letting go through the hinges of your jaw, in the cheeks and anywhere else.
7 Flatten your tongue against the roof of your mouth.
8 Let go.
9 Feel yourself letting go from the roots of your tongue. Feel your tongue widening and softening.
10 Stare hard, then screw up all your eye-muscles, eyelids, the whole upper part of your face.
11 Let go.
12 Feel the muscles of your eyes letting go. Let your eyelids close gently if that is easy. Feel the weight of your eyeballs.
13 On one in-breath, tighten neck, jaw, tongue and eyes. Don't hold.
14 Let go on the out-breath.
15 Check through on successive out-breaths. Feel what is, or is not, letting go in your neck (one out-breath), your jaw (one out-breath), your tongue (one out-breath), your eyeballs (one out-breath) and all four at once (several out-breaths).

LYING

Make sure you are comfortable, with your spine as straight as possible (not flattened into the support, not twisted), your elbows not touching your ribs, your feet falling out to the sides.

1 Tighten your neck very slightly, just enough to feel it.
2 Let go.

3 On the out-breath, feel the letting-go. Next out-breath, sink into the weight at the back of your neck.
4 Tighten through the hinges of your jaw, just enough to feel.
5 Let go. Have your teeth parted.
6 Let your jaw sag. On one out-breath, let go more through the hinges of your jaw.
7 Stick your tongue out as far as you can and stretch it.
8 Let go. Put your tongue onto the lower jaw but don't hold it there.
9 As you breathe out, let go from the roots of your tongue.
10 Open your eyes wide and stare hard.
11 Stop staring. Let the eyelids drop together if that is natural.
12 As you breathe out, feel the weight of your eyeballs.
13 As you breathe in, tighten neck, jaw, tongue, eye muscles, just enough to feel a little tension. Only do this once.
14 As you breathe out, let them all go.
15 Keep breathing naturally and, on every out-breath, keep letting go in your neck, jaw, tongue and eyes.

DAY ELEVEN THE PELVIS

SITTING IN AN EASY CHAIR

1 Tighten your buttock muscles and pull in your stomach muscles. See what else tightens.
2 Let go.
3 Feel the difference. Tighten once or twice more if necessary. Make sure you let go everything that has tightened and then let go a bit more. Check your stomach muscles, spine, groin, thigh muscles and jaw.

LYING

1 Tighten minimally in your buttock muscles and hip joints.

Keep doing it until you know exactly what happens, but only tighten as little as possible to feel.

2 Let go.

3 Feel through your hip joints. Each time you breathe out, let go a bit more in the hip joints. Feel the whole weight of your pelvis as you breathe out. Check that you are not holding your stomach in. Let go in the small of your back. Let go everything inside your pelvis.

DAY TWELVE THE KNEES

STANDING

First, stand in your usual posture. Notice if you stand with more weight on one leg and, if so, what follows from that. Now, stand with your feet hip-width apart and your weight equally on both feet, which should be parallel.

1 Tighten your knees as much as you can. Notice what else tightens. Pull your knee caps up and feel where the tension spreads to.

2 Let go and stand with your knees slightly bent.

3 Feel the difference . . . in knees, thigh muscles, hips, spine, calves, feet . . . anywhere else?

LYING

1 Tighten in your knees, by pressing the backs of your knees towards the support. (This need not be a big movement, but do it until you are sure what is involved.)

2 Let go, letting your knees roll outwards.

3 Feel. Give yourself several out breaths to concentrate on the feeling of letting go in your knee joints. If you find it hard to feel two places at once, feel your left knee joint on one out-

breath, your right knee joint on one out-breath, both knee joints on one out-breath . . . and so on.

DAY THIRTEEN THE ANKLES

SITTING IN AN EASY CHAIR

1 Bend your feet up at the ankle (the opposite of pointing the toes). Feel the tension in your ankle joints.
2 Let go. Have your feet flat on the ground.
3 Feel your ankle joints letting go. As you breathe out, concentrate on your ankles and notice where else lets go.

LYING

1 Point your toes upwards, but not hard. Just move enough to feel your ankle joints working.
2 Let go.
3 Let your feet flop out to the sides, feeling the weight at the heels. Make sure you're not using the ankle joints. On the out-breath keep feeling any sensations in the ankle joints and anything that follows from that.

DAY FOURTEEN THE FEET

SITTING IN AN EASY CHAIR

1 Screw up your feet. Tighten all your toe joints, the arches, your insteps, the skin over the soles of your feet.
2 Let go before you get cramp.
3 Have your feet flat on the floor and feel the letting go in the soles of your feet. As you breathe out, pay special attention to your insteps, your arches, your toe joints. On one out-breath, see if you can feel all the way to the tips of your toes.

LYING

1 Tighten minimally in your feet. Rather than doing a lot, just notice what you do to express tension in the feet.
2 Let go.
3 Let your feet fall out to the sides. Give yourself several out-breaths to feel as much as possible in the soles of your feet, then transfer your attention to your insteps. Then think your way down from ankles to the tips of the toes, doing your feeling (but no moving) on the out-breath.

N.B. If you can't feel your toes, it doesn't help to twiddle them. Once you have tightened and let go, don't move again but just feel the absence of feeling. This does not apply to cramp. Move if you are in agony, but only then.

DAY FIFTEEN RECAPITULATION DAY

SITTING IN AN EASY CHAIR

1 Tighten buttocks.
2 Let go.
3 Feel all buttock muscles and stomach muscles letting go.
4 Stick your legs straight out in front of you and tighten the knees. Pull your knee caps upwards.
5 Let go. Have your feet flat on the floor and your knees falling outwards.
6 Feel your knee joints letting go as you breathe out.
7 Keep your heels on the ground and point your feet upwards. Feel the strain in the ankle joints.
8 Let go and have your feet flat on the floor.
9 Feel the letting go through your ankles.
10 Screw up your feet.
11 Let go and have them flat on the ground.

12 One out-breath, feel the soles of your feet (one first, then the other, then both, i.e. three out-breaths, if you like). The next out-breath, feel the ankles. The next out-breath feel your toes.

13 Keep bringing your mind back to your breathing. When you're ready, feel the buttock muscles on one out-breath, the knees on the next out-breath, the ankles on the next, the feet on the next, and then for several out-breaths, feel yourself letting go from your hip joints down to the tips of your toes.

LYING

1 Minimal tension in your buttocks, hip joints, stomach muscles.
2 Let go.
3 Feel.
4 Tighten your knees slightly.
5 Let go. Your knees should be very slightly bent and rolling outwards.
6 Feel.
7 Tighten slightly in your ankle joints.
8 Let go.
9 Feel.
10 Tighten your feet slightly.
11 Let go.
12 Feel.
13 Take your attention to the breathing. Give yourself time to feel every phase, then on the next series of out-breaths, let go a bit more in your hip joints. When you've let go there as much as you can, transfer your attention to your knees. On the next set of out-breaths, let go through your knee joints. Feel all there is to feel. Is the skin softening at the backs of your knees? Are you holding up your knee caps? Can you let go any more in the muscles above your knees? When you've given the knees as much attention as they need, transfer your

attention to the ankles. Feel the letting go in your ankle joints on the next set of out-breaths. Then your feet. As you breathe out, feel the skin on the soles of your feet, your insteps, your toe joints, the tips of your toes. Then, the next set of out-breaths, join them all together. As you breathe out, let go from your hip joints to the tips of your toes.

DAY SIXTEEN THE BREATHING

SITTING IN AN EASY CHAIR

1 Get comfortable and become aware of your breathing. Don't alter it, but follow the pattern. Be sure you know where you breathe from.
2 Put one hand on your chest and one on your stomach. As you breathe in, the top hand should rise. As you breathe out, the bottom hand should rise. If this does not happen, don't worry or try to force it. Instead, notice what does happen. Put your hands down.
3 Do one extra deep breath. Start by breathing out right to the depths of your lungs. Let the lungs fill up naturally, then go back to normal breathing. Notice what you felt. Don't do that often.
4 When you are back to normal breathing, feel it. Be aware of the whole body when you breathe in, when you breathe out. Be aware of the pauses, the bits you miss out, the bits you linger over. Keep taking your mind back to your breathing.

LYING

1 On the in-breath, tighten your fingers, wrist, elbows and shoulders.
2 On the out-breath, let go everything you tightened.
3 Repeat not more than once.
4 Next in-breath, tighten your neck, jaw, tongue and eyes.

5 Let go on the out-breath.
6 Do it again, if you need to feel what happens.
7 Next in-breath, tighten your buttocks, knees, ankles and feet.
8 Let them all go on the out-breath.
9 Repeat if necessary.
10 Go back to normal breathing. Feel the letting go as you breathe out: one out-breath feel fingers; one out-breath feel wrists; one out-breath feel elbows; one out-breath feel shoulders; one out-breath feel neck; one out-breath feel jaw; one out-breath feel tongue; one out-breath feel eyes; one out-breath feel buttocks; one out-breath feel knees; one out-breath feel ankles; one out-breath feel feet. Several out-breaths feel the whole lot.
11 Go back to just following the breathing when you have felt all the letting go you can. Don't worry if you feel some parts more than others.

N.B. Concentration is bound to be a problem. You've probably reached a stage when it's a good idea to record this or get someone to read it to you. If you prefer to read it first and then do it, it doesn't matter that much if you get it wrong. The important thing is for you to feel for yourself. Don't blame yourself if you lose the thread. Just keep taking your mind back to the breathing without blaming yourself.

DAY SEVENTEEN STRETCHING: HANDS, ARMS AND SHOULDERS

SITTING IN AN EASY CHAIR OR LYING

Choose whichever position you find gives best results. Make sure you are comfortable, with your fingers resting on the support or your lap, not touching each other.

1 Stretch your fingers: both lengthen them and part them from

one another as much as possible. Feel the stretch in the palms of the hands.

2 Stop stretching. Put your hands down with the fingers gently resting on something. Don't hold them in any position. Just let them drop.

3 Allow yourself to feel as much as you can in your finger joints. Don't forget your thumbs. Feel what's happening in the palms and backs of the hands as well. Be completely aware of your hands on each out-breath. If you can't feel much, do one out-breath and feel each finger in turn (each joint if you prefer). If you split them up, do one out-breath and feel your whole hand at the end. Always do both sides equally and end by doing them both together, even if you can't feel a thing.

4 Widen your elbows. Stretch them away from your body.

5 Stop stretching.

6 Feel what's happening in your elbow joints on each out-breath.

7 Pull the shoulders down,

8 Stop pulling.

9 Make sure you're not using the shoulder joints any more. Let them come to rest and feel. On each out-breath, allow yourself to let go a bit more through your shoulder joints. Don't *do* it. *Feel* it happening as you breathe out.

10 On the next set of out-breaths, let go from your shoulder joints down to your finger tips.

DAY EIGHTEEN STRETCHING: HEAD, NECK AND FACE

SITTING IN AN EASY CHAIR OR LYING

1 Push your head into the support.

2 Stop pushing. Make sure you are using no neck muscles.

3 Feel. Give your whole neck a chance to let go as you breathe out. Check that you are not tightening in the top of your spine, your tendons, your throat and the skin over your throat.
4 Keep your lips together and pull your lower jaw downwards.
5 Stop. Let the jaw sag.
6 Feel through the hinges of the jaw as you breathe out.
7 Roll your eyes and raise your eyebrows. Frown, blink and repeat.
8 Close your eyes gently and let your facial muscles go.
9 Feel the letting go in the upper part of your face and up over the scalp. As you breathe out allow your facial muscles to sag.
10 Feel the weight of your whole head on the out-breath. Check that you are not using any eye muscles, face muscles and any muscles inside your mouth or over your cheeks, or in your jaw or neck.

DAY NINETEEN STRETCHING: LOWER PART OF THE BODY

SITTING OR LYING

1 Push your pelvis into the support.
2 Let go.
3 Feel.
4 Widen your knees.
5 Stop and let your knees roll outwards.
6 Feel through your knee joints.
7 Point your toes.
8 Stop.
9 Let your feet fall outwards and feel.

10 Take your mind to the breathing and give yourself time to feel it. When you're ready, on the next three out-breaths feel the weight of your pelvis. The next three, feel right through your knee joints. The next three, feel the weight of your feet.

DAY TWENTY RECAPITULATION DAY

SITTING OR LYING

1 Lengthen and widen your fingers.
2 Let go.
3 Feel.
4 Widen your elbows.
5 Let go.
6 Feel.
7 Pull your shoulders down.
8 Let go.
9 Feel.
10 Push your head into the support.
11 Let go.
12 Feel the weight of your head.
13 Pull your lower jaw downwards.
14 Stop pulling.
15 Feel your jaw sagging.
16 Roll your eyes and raise your eyebrows.
17 Stop and close your eyes gently.
18 Feel the weight of your eyeballs.
19 Push your pelvis into the support.
20 Stop.
21 Feel the weight of your pelvis.
22 Widen your knees.
23 Stop.

24 Feel all your leg muscles.
25 Point your toes.
26 Stop.
27 Feel your feet flopping out to the sides.
28 Take the mind to your breathing. Feel your whole body letting go on the out-breath.
29 Be aware on the out-breath, of all the parts you have stretched.
Three out-breaths, feel your fingers.
Three out-breaths, feel your elbows.
Three out-breaths, feel your shoulders.
One out-breath, feel from shoulders to fingers.
Three out-breaths, feel the weight of your head.
Three out-breaths, feel your jaw sagging.
Three out-breaths, feel the weight of your eyeballs.
Three out-breaths, feel the whole of your head.
Three out-breaths, feel the weight of your pelvis.
Three out-breaths, feel your knee joints.
Three out-breaths, feel your feet flopping off the ankles.
30 As you breathe out, be aware of your whole body.

N.B. This looks very precise and, if you like things precise, there's no reason why you shouldn't follow it to the letter. If you don't, remember it's only a rough guide. As soon as your body has got the feel, you can invent your own.

DAY TWENTY-ONE THE WHOLE BODY: TIGHTENING AND STRETCHING

SITTING OR LYING, BUT PREFERABLY LYING

1 Tighten in your hands; the least possible to feel it.
2 Let go.

3 Feel.
4 Stretch your hands (all fingers as well as the palms of your hands).
5 Let go.
6 With your finger tips resting on something, feel yourself letting go more and more in your finger joints and palms of the hands.
7 Tighten your elbow joints, just a little.
8 Let go.
9 Feel.
10. Widen your elbows from the body.
11 Stop all movement in your elbows.
12 Feel through your elbow joints.
13 Tighten in your shoulders, as little as possible.
14 Let go.
15 Feel.
16 Pull your shoulders down.
17 Stop.
18 Feel the letting go through your shoulder joints.
19 Arch your neck very slightly.
20 Stop.
21 Feel in your neck joints.
22 Extend the back of your neck.
23 Let go.
24 Feel right through your neck.
25 Clench your teeth. Tighten your tongue.
26 Let go. Let your tongue sink.
27 Feel.
28 With your lips together, pull your lower jaw down.
29 Stop.
30 Feel through the hinge of your jaw, roots of the tongue, lips, skin over the cheeks and skin inside your mouth.
31 Screw up your eyelids.
32 Let go.

33 With eyelids gently closed, feel the eye muscles letting go.
34 Open your eyes wide. Roll them once round each way. Then blink.
35 Allow your eyeballs to drop back down into the sockets.
36 Feel the weight of your eyeballs.
37 Tighten your buttock muscles.
38 Stop.
39 Feel the letting go through your hip joints and base of your spine.
40 Push your pelvis into the support.
41 Stop.
42 Feel the weight of your pelvis.
43 Tighten your knee joints. Pull your knee-caps up.
44 Let go.
45 Feel what is letting go (and what isn't) in your knees.
46 Roll your knees outwards.
47 Stop when they are comfortable.
48 Feel the muscles above your knees slackening and the skin behind your knees softening.
49 Point the feet upwards.
50 Let go.
51 Feel yourself letting go through your ankle joints.
52 Point your toes.
53 Let go. Let your feet fall outwards.
54 Feel your feet falling away from the heels.
55 Observe your breathing.
56 Feel your whole body letting go on the out-breath. Keep feeling.

Allow yourself a maximum of half an hour. If less, make it a definite time and stick to that. If you get bored in the middle, come back to being aware of your breathing before you stop. Check once a week to see if you can feel a difference between relaxing and just lying there.

DAY TWENTY-TWO THE WHOLE BODY: FEELING THE LETTING GO

LYING

Feel what happens as you settle. Do you need to tense? Do you need to stretch? If so, do whatever you feel is necessary for you to feel the letting go. Check through the body for pain or tension. Be aware of your weak areas. Also be aware of the places where you can let go easily.

Come back to your breathing and watch it. Give yourself time to watch it in more detail. Again, be aware of weaknesses and strengths. Pleasure? Fear?

1 Feel the weight of your whole body on the out-breath. Keep on allowing the body to sink as you breathe out until you have felt all you can.
2 Transfer your attention to the tips of your toes. On each out-breath, feel what's happening there. If you feel nothing, don't try to feel. Just be aware of what's there.
3 Spread that awareness to your insteps and soles of your feet, still doing your feeling each time you breathe out.
4 When you're ready, extend your awareness to your ankle joints and calf muscles. Keep checking what you actually feel, not making it up.
5 Then your knees. Allow yourself to feel what's happening in the knee joints as you breathe out.
6 Thighs, groin, up to hip joints. Keep feeling the letting go as you breathe out.
7 Then be aware of the weight of the pelvis. Give yourself as long as you need to feel what's going on inside the pelvis.
8 Small of your back, the back of your waist and tail bone area. Feel the weight there as you breathe out.
9 On up the spine, feeling any dead patches, feeling the weight

of your whole back, and letting your torso sink on the out-breath.

10 Feel the front of your body too. As you breathe out, feel the skin softening on the front of your body.
11 See if you can let go any more between your ribs, in your lungs themselves, in your solar plexus.
12 Think of your shoulders. Do just one extra deep out-breath at this point and let go a bit more in your shoulders.
13 From the shoulder joints, let go down your arms: your biceps, elbows, forearms and wrists.
14 Still on the out-breath, let go down your arms from your shoulders to your finger tips.
15 The neck: on each out-breath, feel the weight at the back of your neck, the tendons at the sides of your neck, and your throat.
16 Up to the hinge of your jaw: breathe out and let go more than you thought you could in the hinge of the jaw.
17 The tongue: allow it to let go from its roots.
18 As you breathe out, feel the weight of the whole head.
19 Be aware of all the facial muscles and see if you can let them go any more as you breathe out.
20 Feel the weight of your eyeballs and the weight behind your eyes. Sink into that on the out-breath.

Stay as long as you can comfortably concentrate on the breathing and on letting go the whole body on out-breath. Then, to come to, start to breathe in a little more deeply. Yawn if you can, and stretch everything, starting with the extremities. Stretch fingers and toes, hands and feet, arms and legs, your whole spine, waggle your jaw gently. Then, roll over on your side and relax again for a moment before getting up.

DAY TWENTY-THREE LETTING GO FROM THE BASE OF THE SPINE

LYING

Stretch your whole body from the spine. Check your posture making sure that the weight falls equally to each side. If your head is supported, make sure your shoulders are on the lower level. Have a cushion under your knees if you have any discomfort in the small of your back. If that does not cure it, have a cushion behind your waist as well. If you still feel pain in the small of your back, have your feet on the ground and your legs bent.

1 Concentrate on the small of your back and push it into the support.
2 Let go.
3 Feel yourself letting go at the back of your waist.
4 Pull in your stomach.
5 Let go.
6 Feel the abdomen expanding on the out-breath. Make sure you're not holding your stomach in.
7 Tighten the buttock muscles and anything else that follows on.
8 Let go.
9 Keep letting go and feeling your whole pelvis.
10 Observe the breathing and follow it. Don't alter it.
11 When you are with your breathing, begin to be aware of the weight of your pelvis on each out-breath.
12 Still on the out-breath, feel what follows on from that. If you don't feel the weight of your pelvis, feel the whole lower part of the body.
13 When you are ready to concentrate, bring all your attention to feeling the bottom joint of your spine. Sink into that point on the out-breath.

14 For the next few out-breaths let go as much as possible in your hip joints.
15 When you've felt as much as you can in the hip joints, let go from there right down both legs: groin, thighs, knees, calves, ankles, soles of your feet and toes.
16 Still feeling on each out-breath, take your attention back to your hip joints. See if you can let go any more at that point.
17 Concentrate on the bottom of your spine. Then, as you breathe out, take your attention up the spine until you reach the joint between your shoulders.
18 Each time you breathe out, feel the whole weight of your back.
19 On the out-breath, let go through your shoulder joints. If there is a connection with the hip joints, feel it.
20 Let go down your arms from your shoulder joints on each out-breath: biceps, elbows, forearms, wrists, hands, fingers and thumbs.
21 Go back to feeling the base of your spine and, from there, up your spine to your neck.
22 On the out-breath, feel the weight at the back of your neck.
23 Feel the weight of your whole head as you breathe out.
24 Let go through the hinges of your jaw, tongue, lips and cheeks.
25 Your eyeballs and behind the eyes. Feel the weight as you breathe out. Feel any connection with the base of the spine.
26 Come back to feeling the letting go from the base of your spine. Feel the whole body letting go from that point.
27 Keep feeling the whole body until you have done enough.

Come to gradually, stretching and yawning. Then roll over on your side. Don't get up until you have stretched everything which you let go.

DAY TWENTY-FOUR LETTING GO FROM THE TOP OF THE SPINE

LYING

1 Lift your head a fraction. Extend the back of your neck. Put it down again.
2 Feel. Give yourself long enough to be sure that you're not using any neck muscles.
3 Push your head into the support, just enough to feel it.
4 Stop pushing and feel.
5 Swallow.
6 Get the feeling of an open throat and let go there.
7 Pull your lower jaw downwards and feel the stretch there.
8 Stop pulling and feel the letting go.
9 Roll your eyes behind closed lids.
10 Stop moving your eye muscles and let your eyeballs drop back in the sockets. Feel the weight of your eyeballs.
11 Feel the weight of your whole head and check that you're not using any neck muscles. If you are, don't do anything. Just allow them to let go. If they don't, be aware of that rather than forcing any change.
12 Pull your shoulders gently down.
13 Stop pulling and feel what happens through your shoulder joints.
14 Stretch your arms and hands gently and widen your elbows.
15 Let the arms come to rest in a comfortable position and feel all the muscles letting go from shoulder joints to finger tips.
16 Push your whole torso into the support.
17 Stop pushing and feel the weight.
18 Push your pelvis into the support.
19 Stop pushing and feel the weight.
20 Extend right down the legs and point your toes gently.
21 Stop stretching and let your legs fall out to the side.

22 Take your attention to your breathing. Follow it. Stay with it or, if you wander, come back to it.
23 When you're familiar with each phase of your breathing, take your mind to the back of the neck and feel what's happening there. Keep feeling at that point as you breathe out. Sink into that point.
24 Spread your attention to the front and sides of the neck. On the out-breath, feel your whole neck.
25 Be aware of the throat. Allow yourself to rest there. As you breathe out, see if you can let go any more in your gullet and roots of the tongue.
26 Still on the out-breath, feel the weight of your whole torso resting on the support.
27 Add the weight of your legs as well. Sink into the places where you touch the support: buttocks, calves, heels.
28 Feel your whole body as you breathe out.
29 Centre your concentration on your neck area – the top joint of the spine. Feel what happens there as you breathe out.
30 From the neck, spread your concentration to cover your whole body. Be aware of your breathing.

Pay attention to the coming to. Allow enough time to come to gradually and fully.

DAY TWENTY-FIVE LETTING GO FROM THE HEAD

LYING

1 Stretch anywhere you want to. Come to rest in a comfortable position.
2 Be aware of your breathing. When you have established that, feel your whole body.
3 Start to concentrate on your head as you breathe out. Feel its weight. Make sure your neck muscles are at rest.

4 Let go more through the hinges of your jaw. Give yourself time.
5 Concentrate on your tongue for the next few out-breaths. Allow it to subside. Feel the letting go inside the mouth.
6 Feel your lips. They will loosen as you relax. And the skin over your cheeks will soften.
7 Move your attention up to your eyes. Feel the skin round your eyes softening.
8 If you are relaxed, your eyelids will not be tightly closed. In fact they may be just open. Feel the weight of your top eyelids.
9 Then the weight of your eyeballs. Allow them to drop back. Notice what you see, if anything, but do not deliberately visualise anything.
10 As you breathe out feel the weight behind your eyes, if there is one. If not, feel the weight of your whole head.
11 Still use the out-breath to sink into the weight of your head.
12 Feel the weight of your body as well. Keep breathing out and feeling yourself sinking into the support.
13 Feel the weight of your head and body as one entity. Every time you breathe out, be aware of letting go from the head.
14 Give yourself about half an hour (no need to time it) bringing your mind back to the breathing and feeling the weight of your body from the head every time your mind wanders.

Come to gradually by yawning and stretching systematically. Stretch your fingers and hands on one in-breath. Breathe out and let go. Then stretch your toes and feet. Then your arms, your legs, the whole of your spine. Then open your eyes and roll them gently. Close them again and roll your head from side to side on the pillow. Stretch your neck. Screw up your eyes and yawn. Roll over on your side. Don't get up until you've relaxed again for a moment.

DAY TWENTY-SIX THE MUSCLES OF SPEECH

LYING

1 Stretch any part that needs stretching and get comfortable, but not so comfortable that you go to sleep.
2 Establish the breathing. Check through the body. On one out-breath for each feel: toes, insteps, soles of the feet, ankles, calves, knees, thighs, groin, hip joints, pelvis, buttock muscles, stomach muscles, back of the waist, spine, shoulder blades, front of the body, shoulder joints, biceps, elbows, forearms, wrists, hands, fingers, neck, jaw, throat, face, eyes, head and the whole body.
3 Take your attention to your head and feel the weight. On the next two or three out-breaths, let your head sink.
4 Concentrate on your jaw. As you breathe out, feel the weight of your jaw bone, your cheek bones and your tongue.
5 Now say something out loud (the first thing that comes to mind or some words that constantly recur to you). Be aware of the feeling of saying them.
6 Say them again very softly, still feeling every muscle that moves in your mouth, jaw, throat, anywhere else?
7 Mouth the words but don't use your voice.
8 Think them.
9 Let them go, along with all other words. Notice if it is possible for you not to think in words. If it isn't, don't lie there trying, but every time you think a word, see if you can feel any tension in the speech muscles. This takes a lot of practice.
10 Keep feeling the breathing and letting go the muscles of your lips, tongue, larynx, jaw.
11 Go back to feeling your whole body letting go. Give yourself several breaths to feel without doing anything.

DAY TWENTY-SEVEN THE MUSCLES OF VISION

LYING

1 Stretch and get comfortable.
2 Relax your whole body briefly, going through and letting go each part on an out-breath.
3 Open your eyes and see whatever you see. Take in the scene in every detail, moving your eyes, but not your head, to get the whole picture.
4 Close your eyes and establish your breathing.
5 See the picture you've just been looking at, as accurately as possible. Cheat, if you like. Open your eyes and have another look. Then visualise the scene in front of you.
6 Let the picture fade. Keep being aware of what you see behind closed lids and sink into it as you breathe out. Don't try to see anything. Give yourself a chance to let go of seeing.
7 When you're ready, imagine a moving object passing across your field of vision. Only do that once, but notice if you can feel the eye muscles moving.
8 As you breathe out, let go the muscles that moved, or let the picture go.
9 Allow yourself to see nothing, if that is possible. Keep letting go of seeing.
10 When you've had enough, start to feel the weight of your eyeballs, of your head, of your whole body . . . and your breathing.
11 Open your eyes. Move no other muscles but the eyelids. Take in what you see. Then roll your eyes and blink. Then stretch your body.

DAY TWENTY-EIGHT PAIRS

LYING

1 Stretch.
2 Take your mind to your breathing.
3 Begin to feel yourself letting go as you breathe out, first in the finger tips.
4 Spread that feeling to the finger joints and the palms of the hands. Still use the breathing. Don't alter it. Just feel it.
5 Feel yourself letting go from your wrists on the out-breath.
6 Take your attention to the tips of your toes and let go there on each out-breath.
7 Spread the awareness to your insteps and soles of your feet.
8 Feel the weight at your heels and your feet dropping away from that point as you breathe out.
9 Now be aware of fingers and toes, palms of your hands and soles of your feet, wrists and ankles.
10 Give yourself time to adjust to feeling in pairs. If it's difficult, do one out-breath and concentrate on the left hand and left foot, the next out-breath, the right hand and right foot, the next, both hands and both feet.
11 Next set of out-breaths, feel the letting go in your elbows.
12 Next set of out-breaths, your knees.
13 Next set of out-breaths, your elbows and knees. Again, do one side first and then the other, if it helps you to feel more.
14 When you are ready, move your attention up to your shoulders and, as you breathe out, let go from there.
15 Hip joints: give yourself time to feel that whole area letting go as you breathe out.
16 Shoulder joints and hip joints: if you feel a much more general area, top of the torso and base of the torso, that's fine. If you feel nothing, that's fine too. Just allow yourself to register what *you* feel.

17 As you breathe out, feel the joint at the base of your neck. Add your whole neck and your throat if you want to.
18 Take all your attention to the joint at the top of your spine. Spread to the back of your waist and the whole sacral area if that comes easily.
19 Put the two together: top and bottom of the spine. Feel them both on the out-breath.
20 Feel the weight of your head on the out-breath. If it comes naturally, be particularly aware of the letting go between and behind the eyes.
21 Feel the letting go between the eyes, the joint at the base of your neck and the joint at the base of your spine.

N.B. These are only suggestions. There is no prize for feeling what I suggest. If they don't work for you, ignore them.

22 Feel your whole body. Give yourself the chance to feel what you feel.
23 Come to gradually. Stretch everything. Yawn. Roll over on your side. Then sit up.

DAY TWENTY-NINE YOUR WEAK POINT

LYING

1 Stretch well and pay particular attention to any special pains or tensions.
2 Establish the breathing and let go the whole body systematically.
3 Be aware of your weak point: the point where you are in pain or tensest, or the point you feel least. Do any exercises to ease that point if you need to.
4 Become totally aware of the breathing, particularly in the region of the solar plexus.

5 Feel yourself taking in energy there and letting go from your weak point.
6 When you have felt all you can in your weak point, spread that awareness to other parts of the body. Allow time to reach the whole body.
7 Feel the body as a whole and stay with the breathing.
8 Go back to being aware of your weak point.
9 Then back to the whole body. Stay as long as you are totally aware of the breathing.

N.B. This should last about half an hour. The idea is for you to invent your own relaxations from now on. Be as specific as the book, but don't become dependent on it.

DAY THIRTY OPTIONAL: FOR PRECISE THINKERS

LYING

1 Exercise all you want, then get comfortable..
2 Focus your mind on your breathing. Follow it.
3 For five out-breaths each, feel the following letting go:
(a) Fingers.
(b) Palms of the hands.
(c) Wrists.
(d) Forearms.
(e) Elbows.
(f) Biceps.
(g) Shoulder joints.
4 Give your mind a rest. Just let it wander and then come back to your breathing. When you are back with your breathing again, check from your shoulder joints down to your finger tips for any tensions. Let go all the way down your arms.

5 For five out-breaths each, feel the following letting go:
(a) Neck.
(b) Jaw.
(c) Tongue.
(d) Face muscles.
(e) Eyes.
(f) Whole head.

6 Let your mind wander if it really wants to. Bring it back to the breathing when you are ready and let go the whole of your head from your neck as you breathe out.

7 For five out-breaths each, feel the following in turn:
(a) The weight of the whole torso.
(b) The back.
(c) The front.
(d) The organs: heart, lungs and whatever else you can feel.
(e) The skin, especially that on the front of the body.

8 Again let the mind wander if it wants to. When you bring it back, feel your breathing and feel the weight of your whole body.

9 For five out-breaths each, feel:
(a) Hip joints.
(b) The small of your back.
(c) The organs inside the pelvis.
(d) Stomach muscles.
(e) Genitals.

10 Give the mind a short rest and then come back to following your breathing.

11 For five out-breaths each, feel:
(a) Thigh muscles.
(b) Knees.
(c) Calf muscles.
(d) Ankles.
(e) Feet.

12 Return to breathing or let your mind wander briefly.

13 For five out-breaths each, feel:

  (a) From your hip joints to the tips of your toes.
  (b) From your hip joints up your spine and across your back.
  (c) From your shoulder joints to the tips of your fingers.
  (d) From your neck to feeling your whole head.
  (e) Your whole body.

14 Then come back to feeling the breathing in every phase.

15 Come to in your own way but allow time to stretch everything and remember to roll over onto your side before getting up.

4

RELAXING FOR PARTICULAR COMPLAINTS

AGORAPHOBIA

Agoraphobia means fear of the market-place, or of the outside world. Agoraphobics fear going out and tend to become gradually housebound. In everyday speech, agoraphobia often includes claustrophobia, technically its opposite. Claustrophobia means fear of enclosed spaces. People who can't get into lifts or aeroplanes are technically claustrophobic. But you have to go out before you can get into a lift or an aeroplane. More than that, it isn't what you're afraid of but the fear in itself that is important in dealing with phobias. It is much easier to move phobias around than to get rid of them. In using relaxation to alleviate phobias we do not go into what caused them, interesting though that may be. It is what you feel *now* and where you feel it physically that are the starting points.

So, think of your most frightening situation and feel, physically, where you feel the fear. Where do you tighten up against it? Be absolutely aware of that place and what's happening there. If you can't think of a physical reaction, or if it's somewhere like the heart, where you have no voluntary control, concentrate on the buttock muscles and base of your spine.

1 Be aware of everything that's happening in the area you are

concentrating on. Are you tightening muscles? Is there pain, discomfort, tension? Explore these feelings and the emotions associated with them.

2 Exaggerate. Tighten all the muscles in your chosen area. Feel the tension.

3 Let go and feel the difference. Make sure you can recognise the difference between tension and relaxation. Don't bother too much about differences in your state of mind. Concentrate on feeling a physical difference.

4 Carry on letting go. Now that you can feel the difference between tensing and letting go, let go as much again.

When you can feel this, combine it with the breathing.

1 Be aware of where you are tense.
2 Breathe in and tighten as much as you can.
3 Breathe out and let go.
4 Next in-breath, don't tighten, but next out-breath, let go. And so on. Keep on letting go on the out-breath for another five breaths. Then, go back to normal breathing and let your mind wander.

Only when you have got used to locating your tension physically and letting it go, come back to your phobia. If it's still as bad, forget it again, but keep on learning to relax. Read Claire Weekes' *Self Help for Your Nerves*. Use her advice in conjunction with relaxation. You will find in time that you have a tool for use in panic situations. When you are sure that you can *feel* the letting go on the out-breath, you only need one out-breath to restore your confidence.

ASTHMA

Asthma is a breathing problem not necessarily brought on by tension, but generally made worse by it. Releasing tension helps.

Start by forgetting all about the breathing. Then:

1. Be aware of tension in any part of your body. Stop everything else except breathing and just watch what you are doing . . . what muscles your are using unnecessarily. If you can't think of anywhere that *you* particularly tighten, concentrate on your jaw.
2. Exaggerate this tension. Clench your teeth, or tighten your tensest part. Feel it.
3. Let go. Feel the letting go. Register the difference.
4. Let go a bit more.

Do this until you get the feel of it. Particularly, get the feel of letting go. Then go through the same routine, using the whole body.

1. Be aware of the body.
2. Tighten every muscle.
3. Let them all go.
4. Let them all go as much again.

If you cough while this is going on, don't worry. Just carry on, but notice what you feel. Don't ignore your coughing, but don't let it stop you. Just be aware of it. If it does stop you, start again.

Practise tightening and letting go as often as you can. Whenever anything reminds you, e.g. whenever you cough, tense and let go the whole body. Then, go on letting go. Do this as often as possible. The minimum is 5 minutes twice a day. Carry on like this for a month before you concentrate directly on your breathing.

When you feel ready to observe your breathing, do it for short times at first. One in-breath and one out-breath is enough. Just get the feel of how you breathe. Do this whenever you remember to. Notice your emotions when you watch your breathing. If they are fear, panic, desperation, don't push yourself. Just watch for a moment, without reacting. Keep coming back for another look.

During this time when you are taking quick peeps at your breathing, keep doing your relaxation practice. Tighten and let go without reference to the breathing. When you're sure you have the feel of letting go, try doing it without the preliminary tightening. Do you begin to notice that you let go on each out-breath? Don't force it. You do this anyway, whether you want to or not. It is more difficult to let go without the help of the out-breath.

Do you like making things difficult for yourself?

EATING DISORDERS: OVER-EATING/ANOREXIA

Naturally, we get hungry when the body needs food and stop wanting to eat when we've had enough. This still happens to a surprising number of people considering how far we are from nature.

Those of us in whom this natural balance has become disturbed, either eat too much or too little. They may even alternate between the two.

We need to regain our natural balance.

The first thing to do is resolve to listen only to what your body wants, not to what your mind thinks it ought to want.

Never eat anything you don't really want.

Never stop yourself eating when you are really hungry.

But, the body may have learnt false appetites and addictions.

Once the balance is upset, it's not so easy to recognise what the body really wants.

For righting the balance, yoga may be useful and relaxation should be used as part of a balanced programme of exercise and relaxation.

For particular moments when you want to go on eating, but you know you've had enough, or you don't want to eat but you know you need to:

1 Recognise your state. Be quite clear that this is a morbid condition. Do you really want to change it?
2 If so, learn to relax, but take sensible exercise too. Then, when you can actually feel the relaxation working and you are sure you can recognise the difference between tension and relaxation in your own body, lie down and *feel*. Don't force your thoughts at all. Just watch what you are thinking. If you are craving food, don't think about food. Watch the mental process of craving, without analysing. Just be aware of the feeling. Do exactly the same if the feeling is aversion to eating.

   Be quite sure you know what you feel. Never mind why. (Both these states of mind are connected with the question 'What do people think of me?'.)
3 When you are quite sure you know what you feel, go right through your body letting go. Feel your whole body. Be aware of what you are doing to it.
4 Keep on letting go on each out-breath. Come back to the feeling. In this relaxed state, you can programme your unconscious with different suggestions if you want to. Before you try this, be quite sure the new suggestions are better than the old.

EYE STRAIN

Many eye complaints are caused by the way you use your eyes. Do you stare fixedly? Blink infrequently? Never use your eye muscles? Read in bad positions or bad lights? Watch a lot of television in a slumped position?

If you have eye troubles which are not cured by wearing glasses, it is worth finding out about Bates' method and doing Bates' exercises. (Bates' *Better Sight Without Glasses* and Aldous Huxley's *The Art of Seeing*.)

Learning to relax the eye muscles is as important as learning to exercise them. Use Bates' 'palming' between each exercise (see p.34). At first you won't feel much, but persevere with palming until you stop seeing anything when you do it. Then you will want to go on.

As well as Bates' exercises, do this twice a day:

1 Lie down and close your eyes. Check through and relax the rest of your body before you concentrate on the eyes. Start by feeling your breathing. Then, on one out-breath, make sure you are relaxing your feet and ankles. The next out-breath: let go in your calves and knees, concentrate on relaxing thighs and groin. Next out-breath, back of your waist and base of your spine. Next out-breath feel your whole torso sinking onto the support. Next out-breath, let go your shoulders. Next out-breath, shoulders and down your arms to your hands. Next out-breath feel your neck letting go. Next out-breath feel the weight of your head.

   Now concentrate on your eyes. On each successive out-breath, feel what is happening in the eye muscles, the eyeballs, behind the eyes. Keep on until you've felt all you can.
2 Screw up your eyelids and the skin around your eyes. Feel that, and release when you've felt all you can. Also, notice what you see behind closed lids. Notice if you go on using your eye muscles after you've relaxed the eyelids.
3 Go back to feeling the breathing and letting go on the out-breath. Check the rest of the body. When it is relaxed, concentrate on the eyes. Feel the weight of the eyeballs. On each out-breath, allow them to sink backwards in the eye sockets.
4 As you go on concentrating on the out-breath, see if you can let go behind your eyes and between your eyes, so you feel the weight between your eyes. Allow yourself to sink into that weight as you breathe out.

HYPERTENSION

Hypertension is abnormally high blood pressure. It is the classic case where orthodox medicine uses relaxation techniques. You can lower your blood pressure by learning to relax and you can prove it.

If you are on drugs to lower your blood pressure and you want to come off them, consult your doctor. You can work out a programme for coming off gradually as the relaxation begins to work. Do not attempt this suddenly or without a doctor's advice. Learn to relax for at least a month before you consider withdrawing from drugs.

If you are not on drugs to lower your blood pressure, relaxation will be more rewarding to learn. You will feel it working more quickly.

1. Recognise your tension. What makes you feel your blood pressure is high? If you only know because some doctor told you, notice what you are doing with your arms and hands. Check your tongue, jaw and neck. Do you hold them in any particular position? Be aware of any particular way *you* have of expressing tension.
2. On one in-breath, tighten all your muscles.
3. On the next out-breath, let them all go. Don't do this more than once. Now go back to normal breathing and check what you feel. Keep feeling and notice the parts you didn't reach. You may not have gone right down to the feet. Perhaps you missed the face? If you want to do it again, do just one in-breath and tighten, one out-breath and let go, and then keep on breathing normally and feeling.
4. On each out-breath, let go a bit more. When you get used to feeling the body let go on the out-breath, you can check through different parts of the body, one for each out-breath. Don't control your breathing in any way. Just feel your muscles letting go as you breathe out.

You can do this several times a day in any position. As well as this, twice a day (say morning and evening), lie flat on your back (or as near flat as is comfortable) and do the same thing for 5 minutes undisturbed.

When you get practised at feeling your muscles letting go, you need to do less tensing in order to feel. At the beginning, you may want to repeat the tensing on the in-breath three times. Don't do more. You'll find there'll come a time when you don't need to tighten in order to feel the letting go. When you reach that point (perhaps at the end of a month?), you should start relaxing for half an hour a day.

Follow the 30-day plan in Chapter 3 of this book.

If you feel you need more exercise, it's worth trying yoga.

Also, take every opportunity to walk.

INCURABLE AND TERMINAL ILLNESSES

These are the ones that make teaching and learning relaxation worthwhile. We are all going to die. It is only a question of how soon and in what way. The sooner we start learning to relax, the better we will be able to cope with any pain, and death itself, when the time comes.

The only condition for learning to relax is being able to breathe.

I will assume that you're lying in bed and that some part of you is in pain. For a start, concentrate on that part. Keep bringing your mind back to your physical condition. If you have no actual pain, feel your whole body.

1 Feel what is happening in your body. Don't exaggerate or dramatise. Just feel. It doesn't matter if you don't know exactly what's happening in scientific detail. Feel what *you* feel.
2 As you breathe in, tighten all your muscles.
3 As you breathe out, let them all go.

4 On every subsequent out-breath, keep letting go. Go systematically around the body, letting go all muscles: hands, wrists, elbows, shoulders, neck, jaw, face, eyes, down the neck, back, front, rib cage, hips, thighs, knees, ankles, feet – the whole body. Feel its weight. Feel all the places where it touches the bed. Sink into the pain as you breathe out. Then go back to feeling the whole body and letting it sink on the out-breath.

Don't concentrate on this for too long at first. Keep coming back to it.

When you've had enough of feeling the body, keep coming back to your breathing. Follow it with your mind. It doesn't matter how unnatural it is, just follow what's there. Go with each breath wherever it leads.

If concentration is the problem, don't let that worry you. Let the mind wander off.

Then bring it gently back to your breathing.

Then let it wander off again.

There will be times when you can't keep your mind on your breathing at all and other times when the breathing comes to you.

At times when you're with the breathing, allow your whole body to sink into the out-breath.

Allow your mind to go where it wants.

But watch your thoughts rather than reacting to them.

INSOMNIA

Insomnia is not being able to sleep. This takes many forms. Some people can't get to sleep. Others drop off easily but wake too soon. Some claim never to sleep at all. The problem is usually not so much lack of sleep as worry about it.

Why does it matter so much whether you sleep?

How much sleep do you believe you need?

People need varying amounts, but it is not so much the number of hours as being allowed to go through the various phases of sleep that is important. This can be done in a short space of time and if it is not done, the body will make up what it needs if it is allowed.

Allowing is the clue. Insomniacs are not allowing themselves to get what they need.

You can cure this quite easily by learning to relax *if you want to*.

Take it in stages:

1 Do you worry about not sleeping? Think of all the time you save. Take up some silent occupation. (Learn a language; take a course: something in which you can make progress.) Never try to go to sleep. *Try to keep awake.*

2 Learn to relax *instead* of sleeping. Half an hour of deep relaxation will rest you as much as many hours of sleep. When you are lying in bed wide-awake (*half-awake won't do*):

   (a) Lie flat on your back and be aware of your position in the bed. Feel exactly where you are putting your head, your shoulders and arms, your torso, your legs and feet. Give special attention to any parts you can't feel. Notice the weight of your body.

   (b) Tighten every muscle in your body. Don't do this for long. A second or two is enough. Stop doing it when you are sure you've felt the tension everywhere.

   (c) Let go. Check right through the body. Are you letting go your toes? Ankles? Calf muscles? Knees? Thigh muscles? Groin? Buttock muscles? Stomach muscles? Small of the back? Lungs? Muscles between the ribs? Shoulders? Biceps? Elbows? Forearms? Wrists? Fingers? Thumbs? Neck? Jaw? Tongue? Facial muscles? Eyelids? Eyes?

   (d) Keep on letting go for 5 minutes. On every out-breath let go a little more. Keep checking through the body and don't let anything distract you. If it does, start again. Persevere. Don't sleep.

3 When you begin to get the feeling of relaxation (maybe after a month of doing it every night, maybe longer) you can use it to induce sleep if you want to.

WARNING: be sure you really want to. Sleep is hard to control, as you know. If you've been starving yourself of it for a long time and now suddenly find you can have as much as you want, you may go the other way and find you never want to wake. You may also find that every time you relax, you fall asleep.

If you still want to:

(a) Get yourself lying in bed and relaxed. Having gone through your relaxation practice, turn over onto your side, if you naturally sleep in that position.
(b) Become totally aware of your breathing.
(c) Now, feel your right foot without moving it. Feel yourself letting go the tip of the right big toe. Feel the nail resting on it. Feel the joint of the right big toe letting go. Feel the joint where the right big toe joins onto the foot. Then turn your whole attention to the next toe. Feel the tip, the nail, the first joint, the second joint, the joint joining the toe to the foot.
(d) Go right through the body like that.
(e) This time, don't stop yourself going to sleep.

But don't let your mind wander off into day-dreaming. Either you're concentrating on letting go or you're asleep.

When you get practised at relaxing, you will notice there are not just two states of consciousness: sleep and waking. There are any number of sleep-related states. Be as conscious as you can of what is happening and of what you are doing to yourself.

LUMBAGO

Lumbago means pain in the lower back. It covers a multitude of pains with different causes which cluster around the base of the spine.

Back pain is often crippling, often caused by an injury, or by many small injuries, resulting from using the spine inefficiently. It is usually helped by relaxation. If tension is a major part of the cause, relaxation may cure it. Relaxation combined with an understanding of how we misuse the spine, often will.

We tend to stand, sit, walk and lift things in ways for which the spine was not designed. (See Wilfred Barlow's *The Alexander Principle.*)

For the early acute stages of back pain, rest is the only answer. To speed the departing pain and to guard against its returning, try the following:

1 Lying on your back, hug your knees and roll gently from side to side.
2 Then lower your legs gently to the floor and relax lying flat on your back.
3 Bend one knee and take the bent leg across the body resting the foot on the floor if it will go without straining. Put it down and do the same with the other leg. If this is easy, do it with straight knees.
4 When you get to the furthest position, relax the whole body.

And now, when you're lying on your back, stay there and get comfortable. Prop yourself up with cushions if necessary. With a really bad back a good position to lie in is with your legs up on a chair or sofa. Your back is on the floor, your thighs vertical, and your calves horizontal and supported.

1 Feel your position. Sink into it. Notice where you feel pain. Sink into that. Take one in-breath and, as you breathe out, concentrate on feeling all you can in the small of the back.

Then, go back to normal breathing. Be aware of any other pain or tension.

2 Exaggerate the tension in the lumbar region, not until it's unbearable; just enough to remind yourself. Be aware of exactly what you're doing to produce that tension.

3 Let it go. Feel the difference. If you have to tighten up again to feel the letting go, only do it once.

4 Keep on letting go. What stops you?

When you have got the feel of tightening, letting go, and then going on from there to let go still more, start to coordinate this with breathing.

Breathe in as you tighten and out as you let go, and then carry on letting go on each subsequent out-breath.

Allow the whole body to let go, radiating out from the small of the back.

Come back and check the lumbar again when you have gone through the rest of the body. Then concentrate on the whole body letting go together from the small of the back.

Whenever you get up from relaxing on your back, make sure you roll over onto your side first.

MIGRAINE

The term migraine originates from a Greek word and means a headache confined to half the head. Even a very severe headache is not necessarily a migraine, which usually has accompanying visual disturbances and sometimes an upset stomach as well. Nobody knows for certain what causes migraine but it is connected with dilation of the blood vessels in the neck.

If you suffer from migraine, or even severe headaches, you are probably aware of the connection between tension in the neck and your headache. So, first roll your neck, gently and slowly.

Drop your head as far towards your chest as you can without

pain, then roll it towards your left shoulder, again stopping short of the really painful bits.

Then, roll it backwards, and then towards the right shoulder.

End up with it dropped towards the chest again.

Now go round the other way.

The point of a neck roll is to ease, so be careful not to roll so far that you pull a muscle.

It also helps some people if they massage the back of the neck gently.

Moving the head gently to and fro, or round and round with your fingers on the bottom joints of the neck can sometimes bring relief.

If you can, get someone else to massage the back of your neck. While you have an accomplice, lie on your back and have your head gently pulled so that the whole of your spine is extended.

All these things help me. But do them very gingerly until you know what you are doing or what is being done to you.

Another practical tip that has helped me with headaches is to massage the temples. If you press the whole area round your temples, you will probably find a sore patch, like a bruise. This often becomes sore before a bad headache. Quite a hard massage in that area often relieves a headache and sometimes prevents it. Another way of knowing when a headache is due is to roll your eyes. If it hurts when you look diagonally upwards, it's time to massage the temples. If your headaches are connected with what you eat, it is also time to stop eating your trigger foods.

Relaxation helps too. It really does. Again, it is cumulative.

Relaxing into a headache may occasionally cure it, but, to get consistent results, you need to start before the headache is at its worst and to make a habit of relaxation.

1 Lie flat on your back or recline. Be comfortable, with your head supported. *Feel* from the inside where you are tense. Particularly, be aware of your neck.

2 Arch your neck. Feel the tension. Feel where it spreads to.
3 Let go. Feel the difference. Be sure you give your muscles and brain time to register that difference.
4 Let go more. Keep feeling what is happening, particularly in the neck and head as you breathe out and let go.

Do this several times a day for short periods. Then do the 30-day plan in Chapter 3.

Headaches have different causes. Relaxation will cure tension headaches (if you persevere). It will improve most migraines and cure some.

Headaches that do not respond to relaxation alone can often be cured by the use of words in conjunction with relaxation (see Herbert Benson's *Beyond the Relaxation Response*).

1 First, relax. When you can feel yourself letting go, establish your breathing. Be sure you can feel yourself letting go on the out-breath.
2 Now, think of a word or phrase which is meaningful or soothing to you, e.g. (for people with religious traditions or interests) Kyrie Eleison, Shalom, Allah, Aum. Or (for people without) Letting go, Peace, One Two Three, No Headache. It doesn't matter what you say as long as you like it and stick to it.
3 Then, relax, keep your mind on the breathing, and every time you breathe out, say your chosen word or phrase. You can say it aloud or silently, or just think it. But keep on until it is as inevitable as the out-breath. Feel the headache as you do this. Don't ignore it. Say the words through the headache, as it were.

Don't expect to succeed the first time. You'll succeed sooner than you thought you would.

N.B. This works so well, that you may be covering up some

symptom you ought to know about. If you use this method a lot, be sure you know what is causing your headache. If you don't, ask a doctor.

NERVOUS BREAKDOWN

You are having a nervous breakdown for a good reason. It is your body's response to intolerable strain. Let it take its course. You have reached a stage now where you can't fight any more, so don't try to fight. This is nature's way of forcing you to relax.

You will be surprised what a short time your breakdown will last if you go with it.

To go with it, indulge yourself. Eat what you like. Sleep when you like. Cry if you want to. Take as much exercise as you feel you want. And teach yourself to relax.

Start slowly, but practise regularly. Do 5 minutes relaxation twice a day for the first week, 10 minutes twice a day for the second week and so on.

In that way, do the plan in Chapter 3. Don't practise for longer than half a hour at a time.

While you are learning to relax, practise going *with* negative emotions (relaxing into them) rather than fighting against them.

It's painful, of course, but it's not as painful as trying to run away.

As you learn to let go your physical muscles, you will find that there is a difference between emotions and their objects, e.g. fear is not the same as what you are frightened of.

Concentrate on the emotion (the actual feeling of fear) and not on the object. Relax into the feeling. Let it do its worst.

When you have been relaxing systematically for 2 weeks, do this exercise every day:

1 Lie down in your most comfortable position and allow yourself to feel. Give yourself time to observe your most

painful emotion. Don't invent or exaggerate. Feel only what's really there.

2 Express that emotion in any way that comes spontaneously. Just do this once. Don't make it a performance or an excuse or an analysis. Just let the expression come, without impeding or elaborating.

3 Let it go. Leave the emotion now and concentrate on the breathing. On every out-breath, let go, physically and mentally. Specially, let go of blame. That includes blaming yourself.

4 Let go more. On each out-breath, let go of something different. Do it physically first, going round the body. Then try letting go of individual grievances, things you have against people, things you crave and grasp at and regret. Stop when you run out of grievances.

A nervous breakdown is a turning point. You are being offered new ways of seeing yourself and the world. You don't have to go back to the old ways.

PAIN

Pain can be temporary or chronic. If your pain is chronic, it is worth taking trouble learning to relax because, when you become skilled, you can live with things that were unbearable before. I'll come back to chronic pain, assuming that you have taken a month to do the plan described in Chapter 3.

Before you learn to relax to cope with pain, here are two warnings:

1 Make sure you know the cause of your pain.
2 Don't stop taking painkillers overnight.

Learning to relax is a gradual business and so should coming off drugs be.

TEMPORARY PAIN

If you haven't learnt to relax beforehand, there's not much you can do about accidents except remember two general rules: the more you tighten against a pain, the worse it becomes. And you will feel more pain if your breathing is hard and shallow.

If your have learnt to relax, you have a tool which is useful in any crisis. When pain strikes:

1 Allow yourself to tighten up, scream, react in whatever way comes naturally to you. There is a kind of natural anaesthetic which will help you through the first few minutes.
2 When you have tightened, make sure you let go all the muscles you clenched. Do not prolong the clench beyond what is natural.
3 Concentrate on the pain and let go in that area as much as possible.
4 Concentrate on the breathing and let go through the pain on each out-breath. Persevere. If it becomes unbearable, give yourself a rest. Tighten up, scream, take painkillers . . . whatever. Then go back to letting go through the pain on the out-breath.

CHRONIC PAIN

Chronic pain is always there. It wears you down. You feel if only you could get a break from it, you could cope with it. It is sometimes worth taking drugs to get that break. When you are feeling strong, observe the pain just as a phenomenon. See if you can separate the pain from your emotions about it.

Use a word or phrase as a sort of cry for help or reminder that it is possible to detach your emotions from your physical pain. It isn't easy at first but it comes with practice.

The Christian 'Lord have mercy' is useful for this purpose because it expresses the sort of emotion one feels in chronic pain. But any word or phrase that has meaning for you will work. It's not what you say that matters. It's keeping on saying it. Then:

1 Get as comfortable as you can and concentrate on your pain. Feel all there is to feel and also be aware of your emotional reaction to the pain.
2 If you want to, express that emotional reaction.
3 Take your attention to the breathing. Breathe from as low down in the lungs as you can comfortably. When you are totally aware of your breathing, begin to let go on the out-breath.
4 On every out-breath say your chosen word or phrase. As you say it, let go through your pain.

Keep on. Do this whenever you can. In fact, only stop doing it when you have to take your attention to something else. If you are lying in bed, there's no reason why you shouldn't do it all day. It may seem boring at first, but persevere through the boredom.

If you have time and perseverance to do this for some time you will find that you go through various well-mapped phases. This practice will work as a painkiller, then you will see it as a crutch. Don't settle down in any one phase. Go on.

PANIC ATTACKS

If you stimulate all the hormones produced in the fight/flight reaction and then don't use them, what you get is a panic attack. It's like lighting a fire and then blocking the chimney.

Your panic attack will strike your weak spot. You may find you can't breathe, feel sick or are sick, sweat, have diarrhoea, tremble, or all these things and others too.

The first thing is to convince yourself that this is a panic attack and not the symptoms of some rare illness. For this, you may need to consult a doctor. When you are sure you suffer from panic attacks, you will probably be told to learn to relax. And if you do, it will work. If you can stop yourself rousing the fight/flight reaction in inappropriate situations, you can stop your panic attacks.

Tackle this first by learning to relax at times when you feel all right. Do the 30-day plan systematically. Be sure you practise every day.

Once you have got the feel of relaxation, use it in everyday life, not necessarily in panic situations, but whenever you remember. Just use a couple of breaths to change gear, as it were. Do this quick routine in four parts:

1 Stop. Watch the way you are creating tension. Observe where you are tense.
2 As you breathe in, tighten a little bit more. Just enough to feel it.
3 As you breathe out, let go all your muscles, particularly let your shoulders drop.
4 On the next out-breath, let go more, particularly in the jaw.

This is known as the 'emergency stop technique'. It has many variations and you can invent your own. Use it early and often.

If, when you have learnt to relax, you still have a panic attack, take some violent exercise as soon as you feel it coming on. Run until you are out of breath, or do whatever is possible in your situation. It's worth taking time off before the panic has you in its grip. It need not be long and, if you learn to relax, the need will soon pass.

After the exercise, lie flat on your back and:

1 Be aware of your breathing. Just watch it until you have got the rhythm, or lack of it.
2 Feel what happens all through your body on the in-breath.
3 Allow yourself to let go on the out-breath.
4 On each successive out-breath let go a bit more. Feel your weight sinking into the support.

You need not spend more than 5 minutes on this whole

routine. Do it as soon as you feel panic or any physical symptom of panic.

PRE-MENSTRUAL TENSION

Pre-menstrual tension and other hormonal imbalances are often treated successfully with relaxation. It is worth finding out if you need any other treatment. (Read Katharina Dalton, *Once A Month.*)

It is possible you are making difficulties for yourself by the way you hold your pelvis.

Stand with your back (i.e. your buttocks and shoulders) against a wall. There is probably an arch at the back of your waist which is nowhere near the wall. Can you get it against the wall by bending your knees? If you go sliding down the wall with the arch still there (which is much more difficult) you are holding your pelvis rigidly in one position and producing constant tension in that area.

To free the pelvis, experiment with a hula hoop, or dance the rumba, or do anything you can think of which is not a duty, to make yourelf move freely from the hip joints.

When relaxing lying down, make quite sure you are not increasing the tension at the back of the waist. Have a cushion under your knees and another at the small of the back, if necessary.

If you are still uncomfortable on your back, turn onto your side. It is more difficult to learn to relax like this because the spine is crooked, but it is better to take longer learning than to increase your tension. If you do decide to lie on your side, make sure all parts of you are supported.

Before you start to relax, screw up your stomach muscles, buttock muscles, thigh muscles, groin, base of the spine, and then let them all go. Wriggle about until you are comfortable.

1 Lie still and feel where you are tense. Be sure you know exactly what you feel.
2 Express that tension . . . in any way you can. If you feel like screaming, scream as loudly as possible if you are alone. Do it once, then have a pause and see if you got to the bottom of the tension. Have another go.
3 Stop. See if you can feel the difference between this and the second stage. If you can't, try again. When you have got the feel of letting go, pause there. Register that feeling.
4 Let go a bit more. If you know what letting go feels like, there's no reason why you shouldn't do more of it. What have you to lose?

STOMACH DISORDERS: INDIGESTION, ULCERS

Stress will attack your weak spot. If you bottle up your emotions, it may well strike you in the stomach. This is because acid that forms in the stomach as part of the fight/flight reaction is not discharged naturally, but eats its way into the stomach lining. To deal with this problem, you need to attack the cause, which is your reaction to stress.

Learning to relax will not cure your ulcer overnight. It will alter your attitude to life, which may prevent you getting another ulcer. The same with indigestion; if you attack the root of the problem rather than (or as well as) killing the pain, you are more likely to hit on a permanent cure.

It is not difficult to alter the way your stomach works by learning to relax. It will take about a month.

Make sure you get some form of exercise that satisfies you. yoga or T'ai Chi would help. Also, eat sensibly and at sensible intervals.

Do the 30-day plan in Chapter 3.

When you can recognise the feel of relaxation, practise relaxing before meals, even if it is only for a minute or two.

Eat more slowly than you used to.

When you have an attack, which will be less often as the relaxation starts to take effect:

1 Take time off to feel. Lie down in the position you usually use for relaxing and make sure you know exactly what hurts. Concentrate on the feeling and feel it as much as you can.
2 Tighten all your muscles for the length of a normal breath. Feel how it affects the pain.
3 Let go all your muscles as you breathe out. Keep feeling what is happening. Breathe normally and relax into the pain on the out-breath. Feel your whole body letting go.
4 Give yourself 5 minutes to concentrate on letting go on each out-breath. Pay special attention to letting go in your stomach.

Letting go into the pain may hurt more at first, but you will quickly get through that stage if you persevere.

If you take pills for indigestion, don't stop them suddenly. Phase them out as the relaxation begins to work.

In everyday life, be aware of emotions you don't express. Allow yourself to feel them. Notice situations and feelings that you avoid including those you are ashamed of and those which you strongly disapprove of in other people. You don't have to express hostile emotions. Just be aware of them.

THROMBOSIS

A thrombosis is a clot which forms in a blood vessel, usually of the leg, heart (coronary) or brain (stroke). But blood can clot anywhere, for any number of reasons. Stress is usually a contributory factor.

Any sort of thrombosis is a sign that you are misusing your body. You are less likely to have another if you change your ways. Learning to relax is one recommended change.

Follow the 30-day plan in Chapter 3. Five minutes a day is enough to start with, but practise every day. Use relaxation in your everyday life as much as possible.

THROMBOSIS OF THE LEG

Take gentle exercise. Walk as much as possible, but not so far at any one time that you exhaust yourself.

Once you have learned to relax, do it for at least half an hour a day but not for more than half an hour at any one time.

When you are relaxing, don't let your mind wander. Bring it back constantly to the clot in your leg. Let go from that point. (If you have had surgery, concentrate on the wound.)

CORONARY THROMBOSIS

However much damage has been done, you can still learn to relax. Don't worry if there are parts of your body you cannot feel or things you are unable to do.

When you have learned to relax, do so for half an hour every day, using the breathing as your focal point. Every time your mind wanders, bring it back to the breathing. Get the feel of allowing the out-breath to relax the rest of the body. Don't be afraid to feel what is happening. The heart is capable of repairing and by-passing damaged tissue if you give it the chance without interfering.

STROKE

You may have suffered a lot of damage or very little. You may find concentration more difficult than you did before. If this is so, it may help you to use counting in learning to relax.

1 Be aware of your body. Feel what you can feel. Think of your body in three parts: Part One – from the waist down; Part

Two – the torso and arms; Part Three – the head. Get used to that division so that you can feel the three separate areas. Don't worry about any parts you can't feel, but be aware of them.

2 Breathe in and count one. Be aware of your pelvis, legs, feet.

3 Breathe out and count one. Let go from your hip joints to your toes, so that you feel the whole weight of your legs as you breathe out.

4 Breathe in and count two. Feel your torso, shoulders, arms and hands.

5 Breathe out and count two. Feel yourself letting go your back, your shoulders, your arms and hands.

6 Breathe in and count three. Feel your head.

7 Breathe out and count three. Let go from the neck. Feel the weight of your head.

Keep doing this until you associate the count of one with the legs, two with the torso, three with the head. Give yourself a rest.

Don't be alarmed if you are particularly aware of your heartbeat while this is going on.

Have a rest, then come back to counting one, two, three for three successive breaths. Let go a bit more on each out-breath.

Now, instead of counting one one, two two, three three on the in-breath and the out-breath, count on the out-breath only. Let go the whole body every time you breathe out. Don't go on so long that you lose count. Keep coming back to one, if you get lost.

Don't alter the pace of your breathing to fit in with the counting.

Keep on until your mind wanders. When you realise this has happened, be aware of your breathing again. Then stop.

TINNITUS

Tinnitus is a noise in the ears, sometimes continuous, sometimes intermittent, sometimes unbearably loud, sometimes background. It is caused by some disturbance or injury in the middle ear. Most sufferers from tinnitus notice that it is made worse by stress.

There is no cure for tinnitus at the moment, but it is usually alleviated by relaxation. Tinnitus brought on by stress will be reduced if you learn to reduce your level of stress. Also, your altered attitude to life will make you more able to live with your tinnitus.

There are two opposed methods of teaching relaxation for tinnitus, but both involve learning to relax. So take a month and work through the plan in Chapter 3.

METHOD 1

While you are learning to relax, learn to distance yourself from the sound in your ears. Do every deep relaxation as though you were hearing the sound through double glazing.

METHOD 2

Relax *into* the sound in your ears. Use it as the central object of concentration. Keep coming back to it. Do this all the time in your daily life:

1. Every time you are aware of the sound in your ears, stop everything else and listen to it. Concentrate on it.
2. Let it do its worst. See if you can make it worse by thinking about it.
3. Relax into it. Lean against it, as it were.
4. Keep bringing your mind back to it and letting go into it.

Try these methods on alternate days. Use the one that works for you.

TRANQUILLISER ADDICTION

You went onto tranquillisers in the first place to counteract the effects of some stress in your life. If you are now addicted, you have three problems where you had one before. They are: the side-effects of the drug, the addiction and the original problem. Take them in order.

SIDE-EFFECTS OF TRANQUILLISERS

These include headaches, depression, twitching, hallucinations, aches, skin disorders, giddiness and many more. On the plus side, they are additional reasons for getting off tranquillisers, and provide motivation. You can be sure they will all disappear. They will also be alleviated by the relaxation which is part of your withdrawal programme.

ADDICTION

In taking a tranquilliser, you are providing your body artificially with a substance which the body produces naturally. So the body stops producing it. But you can come to rely on the sense of tranquillity, which you can no longer produce naturally. You need to find other ways of producing it. Learning to relax is such a way.

But there is a drawback. Because of the action of the drug, you won't feel much happening when you first start to learn to relax.

You have to carry on in faith at first.

Don't be in a rush to stop taking the drug. Plan your withdrawal in consultation with a doctor.

If you have decided to give relaxation a try, don't go in for the sort of programme which gets you off one drug and onto another.

Go to yoga classes if you possibly can. Yoga won't get you off tranquillisers overnight, but it will build up the sort of physical and mental strength which, in time, will make outside help unnecessary.

At the same time as the yoga, not just at the end of each yoga class, learn to relax.

Give yourself a month, while you are still on the drug, to do the 30-day plan in Chapter 3. As well as the relaxation you do every day, so this several times a day:

1 Stop what you are doing and recognise your condition. Be very specific. What side-effects are you feeling at this moment? Where in the body do you feel it? What do you feel?
2 Exaggerate whatever you feel. Feel it more. Concentrate on it.
3 Let it go.
4 Keep on letting it go.

Do this every time you think about your health or your state of mind, every time you feel like taking a tranquilliser, every time you do take one, or feel its effects.

THE ORIGINAL PROBLEM

When you are off tranquillisers, you may find the original problem has solved itself or is no longer so bad. Tranquillisers are for short-term emergencies and these do pass.

If the problem is still as bad as ever, apply relaxation to the problem in the same way as you used it on your addiction.

If it is a question of accepting something unbearable, try relaxing into the pain instead of resisting it. Let it overwhelm you and do its worst. See what happens. It can't be worse than running away.

5

RELAXING IN PARTICULAR CIRCUMSTANCES

COUNSELLING

The problem in any work of this kind is becoming so involved in the troubles of your clients that you have nothing left to give. This must happen to any good counsellor. There are many problems where the only help you can give is to suffer. Relaxation, when you have mastered it, is a help because it will replenish your strength. This does not happen through any effort of yours, but through not making an effort. You become a channel. All you have to do is not to block the energy flowing through you. You don't have to hold any metaphysical theory to feel this.

If you get depleted by other people's suffering, it's worth taking a month to do the 30-day plan in Chapter 3. It doesn't take long each day.

You will reach a stage when, if you sit down and let go, you feel all your muscles relaxing without having to go through any set routine. Don't stop relaxing regularly every day when you reach this stage, but you can stop the tensing and letting go.

Once you have got the feel of relaxing lying down, you can do it in any position. If the spine is straight, you will feel it working. But take half an hour a day and do nothing else. Concentrate on your breathing.

Every time your mind wanders, bring it back to your

breathing. Don't rigidly exclude the thoughts that arise. Let them come and watch them as you watch your breathing.

The problem of pain – other people's, other animals' – has never been solved. Relaxation doesn't solve it, but it does give you a breathing space. You can distance yourself from the pain of the world for long enough to sort out what you can help and what you have to bear.

Anything you can help, you then put all your energy into. Anything you can't help, you endure. There are two ways of enduring this (fight and flight) and, naturally, the mind alternates between them. Because the subject is so painful, one is liable to hold up the natural process.

One is very liable to suppress one's pain at pain one can do nothing about. But this is self-destructive. If, having learned to relax, you can relax into it, you will find that the natural swing of the perceptions will make you suffer as much as you can bear and then go on to some other state of mind. If you avoid that suffering, it takes over later, with explosive vigour, and your whole life becomes suffering.

So, when you see a familiar pain approaching:

1 Recognise that here is the point where you usually duck and run. Become more aware of your mental processes, so that you notice these moments when you instinctively avoid a subject coming.
2 Meet it head on. Really feel it, just for a second. Allow yourself to feel, and watch the feeling. You don't have to go on compulsively hurting yourself. What you are watching is the feeling, not its object.
3 Allow that feeling to pass. It will anyway. No feeling is permanent. If there is an element of guilt at not suffering, be aware of that too. Be completely familiar with your mental processes. Don't let them fool you.
4 If there is anything you can do, do it now. If not, keep on letting go.

DRIVING

Driving is a stimulating occupation for those who enjoy it and nerve-racking for those who don't. Both groups can benefit from learning to relax. Tension arises particularly in the neck, eyes and thigh muscles.

If you drive all day, it is a good idea to do a neck roll every time you stop. Also, alter the focus of your eyes: blink and look at something close, blink and widen your gaze to take in your whole field of vision, blink and look at the close object . . . and so on. Go for a short walk too.

Drivers who get pins and needles in the hands are tensing the base of the neck. As you are driving, notice how you hold your head. Is it jutting forward, putting all the strain on the joint at the base of the neck? Do you have to do this?

Do you drive with your shoulders held up?

Do you use more leg muscles than you need?

Long-distance driving can be made into a more relaxing occupation by letting go all but the essential muscles on each out-breath. You can also make it safer. When you are relaxing, your mind is in the present. You are much less likely to drive around in a trance.

For traffic jams, take three deep breaths:

1 Breathe in and tense very slightly all over.
2 Breathe out and let go and register the difference. Are you more relaxed now than your normal driving state?
3 Breathe in and feel without tensing.
4 Breathe out and let go your shoulders and down your arms.
5 Breathe in and feel yourself taking in energy.
6 Breathe out and let go in the neck and jaw.
7 Go on for as long as the traffic jam lasts, feeling your whole body letting go on the out-breath. Keep bringing your mind back to the breathing. Be in the present.

For nervous passengers:

Relax with your eyes shut.

Looking out of the side of the vehicle rather than the front helps a lot too.

ELDERLY

If your life is full of aches and pains and boredom, at least you have time to learn to relax. It is not too late.

Take the aches and pains first. Unless the pain is acute, it is a good idea to exercise stiff and aching joints. Keep moving as much as you can, without major exertion. Make sure that your finger joints, knees, spine all get regular exercise. Relax each part you have exercised. Yoga will help a lot, but don't be ambitious. You are not aiming to change your condition but to make the best of it.

Practise deep relaxation as often as you have the time. Several short sessions a day will add up. If you have time for long sessions, so much the better:

Lie, or sit in a chair, but have your whole back and head supported. Have your elbows wide from your sides.

Feel the weight of your whole body.

Take time to get used to the feel of your breathing.

When you are in touch with the natural rhythm of the breathing:

1 Feel the weight of your head and the weight behind your eyes on the out-breath.
2 On successive out-breaths:
   (a) Let the lower jaw sag.
   (b) Let go in your neck.
   (c) Feel your shoulders. Feel the weight.
   (d) From the shoulders, feel all the muscles down your arms letting go.
3 Feel yourself letting go in the fingers and the palms of your hands as you breathe out.

4 For the next two or three breaths, check the relaxation in your head, neck, shoulders, arms and hands. If you still feel any tension, do a few more out-breaths paying special attention to the places where you are still tense.
5 When you're ready, start to feel the weight of your torso as you breathe out. Go on until you've had enough.
6 The next series of breaths, feel the front of your body letting go. As you breathe out, feel your skin softening.
7 When your torso is as relaxed as you can get it, begin to concentrate on your hip joints. Let go through the joints as you breathe out.
8 As you breathe out, let go from the groin to the thigh muscles.
9 Now concentrate on your knees. Make sure that you're not tightening the muscles above your knees, or the skin at the backs of your knees. Give yourself two or three out-breaths to let go from your knees.
10 Then, as you breathe out, feel your calf muscles letting go.
11 Then concentrate on your ankles. Feel the weight of your feet. Let them flop.
12 Next set of out-breaths, concentrate on your feet. Let go in your toes, insteps and soles of your feet.
13 Keep concentrating on the breathing and feel your whole body. Go on letting go for as long as you have time or concentration.

Do this at least twice a day if you have time. For instant relaxation, do just three deep breaths:

1 Breathe in and tighten all muscles very slightly.
2 Breathe out and let go all muscles.
3 Breathe in and feel any tensions without exaggerating them.
4 Breathe out and let go in your shoulders and down your arms.
5 Breathe in deeply and feel yourself taking in energy.

6 Breathe out and let go in your neck and jaw.

You won't feel anything the first time, but keep doing it. Feel what happens at the base of your spine when you have let go all you can in the shoulders and neck.

Relaxation is something you can practise at any time, e.g. when you are awake in the night, and it is cumulative. It is always worth doing a little, even if you feel no benefit at the time.

EXAMINATIONS

The first thing to realise about examinations is that they are not important. The results are important, since people set such store by qualifications. But the examinations themselves bear no relation to your intelligence and not much to your knowledge. Passing examinations is a game with rules. If you want the qualification, you play the game.

So learn the rules and, if you are liable to panic, learn to relax.

On the day, relax before you go into the examination. Take 10 minutes and:

1 Lie down in your habitual relaxing position. Forget all about the examination. Just be aware of your physical state and where you are tense. Concentrate all your attention on your tension.
2 Tighten in the least possible way – just enough to feel the tension. If you are not tense anywhere in particular, induce a little tension in all your muscles.
3 Let go as much as you can and feel the difference.
4 Use the out-breath to let go a little more. Be sure you recognise the feeling of letting go, so you have only to be aware of breathing out and you will feel yourself letting go.

When you are in the examination room, if you get stuck or feel panicky, take two deep breaths. On the first out-breath, drop your shoulders and relax right down your arms. On the second out-breath let go your jaw, neck, throat.

GARDENING

Gardeners have physical and mental problems too, although non-gardeners tend to be sceptical about this. Physical problems collect in the back and neck. Both spring from too much bending forwards.

Pain at the base of the spine can be alleviated before it gets too bad by bending the spine the other way. Stand upright with the feet hip-width apart, hands on hips and bend backwards from the waist. Don't hold the extreme position, but bounce backwards several times with knees slightly bent. Do this often if you are stooping, turfing, pruning low shrubs etc.

Pain in the neck (leading to numb fingers) and head troubles from bending forwards are best counteracted by lying flat on the back and relaxing deeply, concentrating on the neck and weight behind the eyes. Do this for short times (about 2 minutes at a time) as soon as you feel these troubles coming on rather than leaving them for a deep relaxation session when the problem is bad.

Gardeners are pitting themselves against nature but, like hunters, they become closer to their prey than to the rest of the world. So hunters end up preserving wildlife and gardeners tend towards a state where they can't pull up another weed. Most gardeners are melancholy by nature, and gardening increases their natural melancholy to the point of despair. If you have reached this stage, but still have to go on gardening, the only thing to do is to break the task down into smaller and smaller units. Do a little digging, a little planting, a little mowing. Relax between each task and don't ignore the messages from your sub-conscious that come up during relaxation.

INTERVIEWS

Interviews are unfair because there are good interviewees, who give a naturally good impression, whether they can do the job or not, and bad interviewees, who ruin their chances, however good they are.

Relaxation can even up life's unfairness to some extent. If you know you are a bad interviewee, it is well worth learning to relax. When you are at the stage when you can feel relaxation working, you can tackle your interview from two directions.

USING DEEP RELAXATION

Relax as deeply as you can. When you are fully relaxed, take your mind to the breathing. Each time you breathe out, feel your emotions about the coming interview. Don't imagine it. Just be aware of your feelings about it. These are just your feelings. They have nothing to do with what may happen in the future. They are conditioning from the past. Notice how you condition yourself. Feel, physically, how this conditioning affects you. What part of the body do you feel it in? See if you can let go any more in that part. Don't be ashamed of being nervous about the coming interview, or pretend you are not. *Just* feel what you feel without fear and without exaggeration. (If what you feel is fear, don't go in for the secondary fear of dreading feeling the fear.) Go back to feeling the breathing and letting go on the out-breath. Let go of emotions too, if you want to.

FOR USE AT THE TIME

Breathe in deeply and feel. Breathe out deeply and let go in the shoulders and arms. Breathe in deeply and feel. Breathe out deeply and let go in the jaw and neck.

NURSING

Nursing breeds many stress problems. Sleep problems and bad backs are common but nurses also find relaxation useful because they can sometimes pass it on to their patients.

It is worth taking a regular half hour (not necessarily the same half hour) every day to learn to relax. It is also worth working out a series of relaxation exercises that you can do on the job.

I will assume that you have done Chapter 3 of this book. When you get to the end of your month, keep taking a regular half hour a day for relaxation. Begin to use relaxation with two opposite aims: to make you sleep and to wake you up.

TO WAKE YOU UP

1 Get a comfortable position and relax in your usual way. When you are as relaxed as you feel you can be, concentrate on the breathing and on the solar plexus. Feel yourself taking in energy every time you breathe in. Still let go on each out-breath.
2 Start to direct the energy which you take in on the in-breath: e.g. breathe in, take in energy at the solar plexus; breathe out, direct that energy to the toes. (Don't *do* anything. Just feel.) Breathe in, take in energy at the solar plexus; breathe out, direct that energy to the calf muscles. And so on. You are not tightening any muscles. You are merely feeling the energy flow through them. Notice any blocks.
3 When you have gone right through the body, direct energy to the whole body, taking in through the solar plexus and directing to the extremities.
4 Stretch well and give yourself time to adjust before you get up.

TO MAKE YOU SLEEP

If you have difficulty adjusting to different shifts, or to having to sleep for short times, use relaxation to help you sleep. If you have to wake at a set time, you can programme your subconscious, as you are relaxing, to wake you when you want.

1 Get into your normal sleeping position. If that is not lying on your back and you've learned to relax lying on your back only, go through your usual relaxation routine.
2 Be aware of your breathing and of feeling your weight on the bed. On each out-breath, feel yourself sinking into that weight. Before you sleep, be completely conscious of when you want to wake.
3 If you are wide awake now, go through each part of the body in great detail. On the out-breath, feel yourself letting go the tip of the right thumb, then the joint of the right thumb, then the knuckle where the thumb joins the hand, then the tip of the right index finger, and so on. Keep bringing your mind back when it wanders. Don't let the worries of the day impinge.

You may find it easier to make a cassette of yourself saying all this. If you do, make sure you have a machine that turns itself off.

RELAXING AS YOU WORK

1 *Lifting.* The general rule for lifting is to use the leg muscles, not to put the strain on the base of the spine. Always bend your knees before lifting a heavy weight, and breathe out as you do so. For lifting a patient in the bed, it helps if both of you are relaxed and do it on the out-breath.
2 *Giving an injection.* Again, it helps if you and your patient are relaxed. It saves time in the long run if you remember to use the out-breath to let go and give the patient a chance to do so too.
3 *Any job you particularly dislike.* Give yourself a chance to relax

before tackling it. Take two deep breaths. On the first out-breath, let go the shoulders. Let them drop and see if they stay down. On the second out-breath, let go the jaw. Make any particular effort on an out-breath.

PERFORMING

Any performer knows that tension can ruin the most brilliant and carefully rehearsed act. Learning to relax well beforehand is half the battle. Half an hour completely undisturbed before a performance is a help if you've already learnt to relax.

If you work in this way, take 5 minutes to relax deeply. Then, feel the breathing. Then stop using your mind: anticipating, rehearsing, worrying. Just allow yourself to be the person you are impersonating or the speech you are going to give. Letting go of inhibitions is a knack which you can learn in relaxing. Many performers use alcohol for the same purpose. Relaxing works as well without being addictive.

If you don't have time to relax deeply, or don't work in that way, two or three deep breaths immediately before a performance can have a similar effect. The sudden intake of oxygen, combined with relaxation on the out-breath, can overcome last minute stage-fright if it is not severe.

If you get very nervous before a performance, it is worth taking time to learn to relax. Then, when you feel the nerves coming on (before you get paralytic) lie down and go through the whole body, systematically letting go. Now, take three deep breaths:

1 On the in-breath, tighten all your muscles as much as you can. On the out-breath let them all go.
2 On the in-breath, tighten just enough to feel the tension in all muscles. Let go on the out-breath.
3 Breathe in and imagine the tension. Breathe out and let go. Keep on letting go on the out-breath.

PREGNANCY

If you go to National Childbirth Trust classes, or any other antenatal preparation, you will probably be taught to relax. Otherwise do Chapter 3 of this book. It is a good idea to learn to relax and to practise it regularly as soon as you know that you are pregnant.

If you get no other form of exercise, be sure you walk two miles every day. Also give yourself 10 minutes twice a day when you do nothing but relax. In those 10 minutes, go through your relaxation routine and, when you are as relaxed as possible:

1 Feel your position. (It doesn't matter what that position is as long as you're comfortable.) Be aware of your whole body. Notice where you are in pain or discomfort, where you tighten.
2 If you have a particular tension, exaggerate it very slightly. If not, tighten all your muscles just enough to feel that tension. Do this tightening only for the length of one in-breath.
3 As you breathe out, let go everything you tightened.
4 Be totally aware of your breathing and don't alter it in any way. Just feel yourself letting go a bit more every time you breathe out. Do this until the 10 minutes is up.

You may be taught methods of breathing for use during delivery which are different from this. That's fine for special situations, but don't think of relaxation as something you need only when you're giving birth. A relaxation technique that becomes part of your everyday life will automatically help you in crises. It will strengthen you every day as well.

SPORTSMEN

Every sport has its special risks and injuries. These are often 'badges of honour' and considered a just cause for pride. However, tension, as well as producing injuries, can also inhibit performance. Every sportsman plays better relaxed. So it's worth learning how to relax in action. The first stage is learning to relax lying down. When you have mastered this, you will approach your sport with less tension. The object then is to maintain this relaxed attitude while playing.

If possible, give yourself 5 minutes deep relaxation before playing. While you are playing, watch which muscles you tighten unnecessarily. When you know you have tensed up, watch your breathing. Even if you are out of breath, you can still relax by letting go on the out-breath. Don't *control* your breathing; just remember to let go as you breathe out.

FOR RUNNING OR ANY SPORT WHERE ENDURANCE IS VITAL

It helps to repeat a word or phrase every time you breathe out.

Also, notice how much effort you are making with your shoulders. In running, only the legs and feet need to work hard.

FOR BALL GAMES WHERE ACCURACY OF AIM IS ESSENTIAL (TENNIS, GOLF ETC)

Concentrate more on the means than the end. You can be too determined to win. While you are playing each shot, relax into the feel of hitting the ball. Concentrate on the ball, on seeing the centre of the ball, rather than letting your mind run ahead.

WAITING

Many jobs involve long periods of waiting interspersed with bouts of violent activity. People who do them often say they don't mind the action. It's the waiting that gets them down.

You can help both the waiting and the action by learning to relax. For the action, you will be quicker off the mark and need less sleep. The waiting can become a positive pleasure.

Start learning to relax during regular waiting periods. Do it at least once a day.

Choose a time when you are likely to have at least half an hour. Having said that, never mind breaking off in the middle of a relax. You are relaxing in order to make yourself more efficient. You can stop at any moment and crack into action.

1 Get a comfortable position, preferably lying down. Tighten all your muscles. Be aware of the area where you are tense.
2 Let go everywhere you tightened. Feel the difference.
3 When you are sure you have felt that difference, keep on letting go from there.

Do this, just taking a minute or two, whenever you feel you wish you were doing something.

When you have an undisturbed half hour every day, do the 30-day plan covered in Chapter 3.

When you are skilled at relaxing, use it in two different ways: a) to gear yourself for instant action; b) to go deeper.

1 *To prepare yourself for action.* Become aware of your breathing and, when you have the measure of it, do two deep breaths. On the first out-breath, let your shoulders go down, your hands unclench, your neck grow longer. On the second out-breath, let your lower jaw sag and your neck relax. Now, act, but calmly. Feel yourself breathing from the depths of the lungs, not from the upper chest. There is no need to force this breathing. Just be aware of it.
2 *To relax more deeply.* When you know you have a long wait ahead, lie down and induce deep relaxation by any means that works best for you. When you are as relaxed as you feel you can be, take your mind to the breathing and feel what happens in your whole body on each out-breath. Be aware of your *whole* body.

Then, follow the breathing with your mind. Don't try to concentrate too hard, or let your mind wander. (It will, but just come back to the breathing every time this happens.) Just stay with the breathing and see where it takes you. Don't *do* anything to alter the breathing. You are observing, not controlling.

This sounds as boring as waiting when you read about it, and there may be times when it *is* boring. If so, watch the boredom. If you do, you will find it is not static. Whatever happens, it will change all the time.

WORK INVOLVING STANDING

It is important, with jobs of this kind, to relax before you start work. Give yourself 10 minutes of deep relaxation, concentrating particularly on the legs and feet.

Wear comfortable shoes. Even a little pressure on the big toe will produce bunions. If you have a tendency towards flat feet, your arches will fall unless you do remedial exercises. High heels will displace bones in the feet. If you place your weight unevenly on your feet (you can tell this by looking at the way your shoes wear), it is worth doing exercises to correct this.

The way you stand and walk may also be producing unnecessary pains in the legs, hips or lower back. Notice if you habitually stand with your weight on one leg, walk with one or both feet turned out or stand with your back arched. (See Wilfred Barlow, *The Alexander Principle.*)

If your legs ache when you finish work, relax by lying with your back on the floor and your legs resting on a chair, bent at the knee at right angles, so your calves are parallel with the floor. You can do exactly the same relaxation like that as flat on the floor. Or use the yoga position for aching legs, i.e. with your back flat on the floor and your legs against a wall and falling out to the sides.

This is quite a severe pull on the hamstring muscles and not suitable for people who do no other leg exercises.

For relaxing on the job, first notice how you walk. Do you tighten your hip muscles all the time or hold your pelvis in one position? Do you lean forwards or backwards? Practise walking much more slowly than usual and check exactly where you tighten.

Notice if you lock your knees when you're standing. Do you grip the ground with your feet? Practise relaxing from the base of the spine and all the way down the legs to the feet while walking, slowly at first. Then, speed it up. Then run. Notice which muscles you are actually using and which tighten in sympathy. Find the way of walking which is most economical for you. Remember to use it under stress.

When the job speeds up, remember to let go on the out-breath. Check on successive out-breaths that you are letting go hips, base of the spine, thigh muscles, knees, calf muscles, ankles, feet.

If your job allows short breaks on your feet, do two deep breaths. On the first out-breath let go in the hips and base of the spine. On the second, let go right down the legs. If you can do this sitting, or lying, so much the better. If you can lie with your legs on a chair and relax totally for a couple of minutes, you will probably be able to go on much longer.

WORKING IN AN OFFICE

MANAGEMENT

Businessmen I have relaxed have been harassed by competition and by being in a perpetual hurry. Successful businessmen obviously thrive on stress, but there is always a breaking point. Indeed, successful businessmen I have known spend much ingenuity in searching out one another's breaking points. So it is important to know your own.

It is important, too, to take exercise; preferably not squash, which is the exercise most businessmen choose. Squash is the physical equivalent of office life. Something which exercises all the muscles in a less brutal way would be more beneficial and something less competitive would be more of a break, mentally. However, if you do choose squash, it's all the more important to learn to relax.

If you choose to learn relaxation, I've no doubt you will master it quickly and be outstandingly good at it. (Don't make the mistake of giving it up because it is too easy.) So when you've mastered it, keep on relaxing. You're just at the beginning when you feel it working. Relaxation is not static. It's more like reaching an underground river. The creative powers you find in yourself through relaxing will change all the time. If they don't, you'll know you've got stuck somewhere.

Give yourself half an hour of relaxing every day, if you can. But balance it by at least half an hour of exercise.

CLERICAL

Secretaries seem to have two main groups of problems: one is connected with the physical positions they have to work in (neck, shoulder and back problems) and the other with stress they work under.

To take the physical first, make sure you sit at the right height. Do a neck roll (once each way) twice a day. Drop your shoulders often if you feel them tensing up. Roll each shoulder backwards in its socket. Shake your arms and hands like a swimmer preparing for a race. You barely have to stop work to do these. You can relax where you sit too.

1 Have your spine straight, feet flat on the floor and hands

hanging at your sides. If your head is jutting forward, adjust it so that it is balanced on the top of your spine.

2 Breathe in deeply. Feel your lungs expanding outwards. As you breathe out, let your shoulders drop as far as they will. Don't force the out-breath, but breathe as deeply as you can with comfort.

3 Breathe in deeply again. Just let your lungs fill up when you get to the bottom of the out-breath. You don't have to make any effort to breathe. Feel the breath moving up from stomach to chest, chest to throat. As you breathe out this time, let go your lower jaw. Feel yourself settling into your seat as you breathe out. Still don't slump, but let your spine rest.

Then go back to work, but keep your shoulders down and move a little more slowly. The time you spend doing this will be soon made up in increased efficiency.

Being bullied at work is not the monopoly of secretaries. Learning to relax does help in coping with it.

When you have got the feel of relaxation, study your reactions until you know exactly what is upsetting you. What can you do about it? What is the worst thing that can happen?

Relax deeply every day and, when you are relaxed, have a look at your problems. Give yourself a chance to know and understand your feelings.

WORKING MOTHERS

Your main problem will be fitting all your commitments into the time available. It is infuriating when people don't co-operate. And everyone around you, feeling short-changed of your attention, is liable to stop co-operating.

Relaxation can help you in many ways. You will need less sleep and feel less exhausted and so have more time and energy to give.

Also, if you are relaxed, you will pass on this feeling to your family and they will be less ready to play up. So find an opportunity somehow, even if it means getting up earlier or going to bed later, of relaxing deeply for half an hour a day. If that sounds out of the question, don't give up the whole idea. Any time spent relaxing is better than none.

As well as deep relaxation, get into the habit of using relaxation in your daily life. Every time you feel irritation or frustration, remember to let go on the out-breath. You don't have to stop what you're doing. Just relax *towards* the object of your annoyance as you breathe out. You will find you can change people's attitudes to you like this. Don't necessarily hide your feelings.

Any time when you can't break off, just stop what you are doing for the length of two breaths.

1 Be aware of the position you are in. Notice where you are tense.
2 Breathe in and tighten very slightly.
3 Breathe out and let go.
4 Breathe in again and feel yourself taking in energy without tightening.
5 Breathe out and let go, particularly in the shoulders.

Go back to what you were doing, moving slightly more slowly than before.

It is as easy to make everyday life a source of relaxation as a source of tension. Either way, it's *you* doing it. If you notice every time you tense up and deliberately let go every time, you can transform the things that were getting you down into sources of strength.

TO PEOPLE WHO LEARN TO RELAX:

Relaxing is the beginning of a journey,
not a static process.
If you keep relaxing, you will develop.
But you can stop relaxing at any time.
It's up to you.

TO PEOPLE WHO DON'T:

This particular method didn't work for you.
It's as likely to be my fault as yours.
Don't be discouraged.
If you want the benefits of relaxation,
try another method.
You'll get it in the end, if you really want it.

APPENDICES

CENTRAL OFFICES OF ORGANISATIONS DEALING WITH SPECIAL PROBLEMS

Acupuncture British Acupuncture Association, 34 Alderney Street, London SW1 4EV (Tel. 01-834 1012)

Alcoholism Alcoholics Anonymous, Redcliffe Gardens, London SW10 (Tel. 01-352 9779 or 01-834 8202)

Arthritis Arthritis Care, 61 Grosvenor Crescent, London SW1X 7ER (Tel. 01-235 2676)

Back Pain Back Pain Association, Grundy House, 31/33 Park Road, Teddington TW11 0AB (Tel. 01-977 5474/5)

Blindness Royal National Institute for the Blind, 224 Great Portland Street, London W1N 6AA (Tel. 01-388 1266)

Counselling Westminster Pastoral Foundation, 23 Kensington Square, London W8 5HN (Tel. 01-937 6956)

Disabled Disabled Living Foundation, 380 Harrow Road, London W9 2HU (Tel. 01-289 6111)

Homoeopathy Homoeopathic Association, 27A Devonshire Street, London W1N 1RJ (Tel. 01-935 2163)

The Back Foundation, Mount Vernon, Sotwell, Oxfordshire (Tel. 0491 39489)

Mental Illness Mind, 22 Harley Street, London W1N 2ED (Tel. 01-637 0741)

Migraine Migraine Trust, 45 Great Ormond Street, London WC1N 3HD (Tel. 01-278 2676)

Multiple Sclerosis M.S. Society, 25 Effie Road, London SW6 1EE (Tel. 01-381 4022)

Osteopathy Osteopathic Medical Association, 28 Wimpole Street, London W1 (Tel. 01-631 5215)

Relaxation Relaxation for Living, 29 Burwood Park Road, Walton-on-Thames, Surrey (Tel. 0932 227826)

Stroke Chest and Heart Association, Tavistock House North, Tavistock Square, London WC1H 9JE (Tel. 01-387 2012)

T'ai Chi 7 Upper Wimpole Street, London W1M 7TD (Tel. 01-935 8444)

Therapies Association for Humanistic Psychology, 62 Southwark Bridge Road, London SE1 0AU (Tel. 01-928 8284)

Tinnitus Royal National Institute for the Deaf, 105 Gower Street, London WC1E 6AH (Tel. 01-387 8033)

Weight Weight Watchers, 11 Fairacres Industrial Estate, Deadworth Road, Windsor, Berkshire (Tel. 01-580 4765)

Yoga Local Education Authorities *or* British Wheel of Yoga, 80 Leckhampton Road, Cheltenham, Gloucestershire

OTHER USEFUL ADDRESSES

Australia Mr J. Chance, 43/16-18 Kings Cross Road, Kings Cross, Sydney, NSW 2011 (Tel. 02 357 3903)

New Zealand Ms Christine Murray, 20 Selwyn Street, Dunedin (Tel. 024 739 567)

USA Prof. A.D. Murray, 508 W. Washington, Urbana, ILL 61861 (Tel. 217 367 3172)

Ms A.L. Rodiger, 801 Broadway, No. 2, New York, NY 1003 (Tel. 212 637 0111)

BIBLIOGRAPHY

The following are classic popular works on relaxation:

Benson, H. (1977) *The Relaxation Response* Fount
Jacobson, E. (1980) *You Must Relax* Unwin
Madders, J. (1979) *Stress and Relaxation* Martin Dunitz
Mears, A. (1970) *Relief without Drugs* Fontana
Mitchell, L. (1977) *Simple Relaxation* John Murray

The books below are referred to in the text under a particular topic:

Barlow, W. (1975) *The Alexander Principle* Arrow
Bates, W.H. (1979) *Better Sight Without Glasses* Mayflower
Benson, H. (1985) *Beyond the Relaxation Response* Fount
Dalton, K. (1983) *Once a Month* Fontana
Hittleman, R. (1971) *Yoga – 28-Day Exercise Plan* Hamlyn
Huxley, A. (1985) *The Art of Seeing* Panther
Iyengar, B.K.S. (1971) *Light on Yoga* Unwin
Rowe, D. (1983) *Depression* Routledge & Kegan Paul
Weekes, C. (1986) *Self-help For Your Nerves* Angus & Robertson

INDEX

Addiction 101-102
Agoraphobia 75 – 76
Alexander Principle, The 86, 117
Anaesthetics 13, 20
Ankles 50
Anorexia 78 – 79
Anti-depressants 20
Arms 54 – 55
Art Of Seeing, The 79
Arthritis 12
Asthma 76 – 78

Back 17, 86 – 87, 109, 119
Barlow, Wilfred 29, 86, 117
Bates, W.H. 34, 79 – 80
Benson, Herbert 89
Better Sight Without Glasses 79
Beyond The Relaxation Response 89
Blood clot 20, 97 – 99
Blood pressure 81
Breathing 53 – 54, 76 – 78

Cassette 9, 112
Claustrophobia 75 – 76
Colitis 11, 17
Concentration 54
Coronary 98 – 99
Counselling 103 – 104
Cramp 27

Dalton, Katharina 95
Driving 104 – 106
Drugs *see also* Anaesthetics, Anti-depressants, Painkillers, Tranquillisers 12, 20, 81, 91, 101 – 102

Elbows 39 – 40
Elderly 106 – 108
Emergency stop technique 94
Examinations 108 – 109

Exercise 14, 21 – 35, 36, 90, 114 – 115, 119
Eyes 34, 46, 69, 79 – 80

Fear 90, 110
Feet 50 – 51, 117 – 118
Fibrositis 12, 17
Frozen shoulder 12, 17

Gardening 109

Hands 37 – 38, 54 – 55
Headaches *see also* Migraine 12, 17, 18 – 19, 20, 87 – 90, 101, 109
Heart attack 98 – 99
Hittleman, Richard 11
Housework 32 – 33, 120 – 121
Huxley, Aldous 79
Hypertension 11, 81 – 82

Incurable illness 82 – 83
Indigestion 96 – 97
Insomnia 11, 83 – 85
Interviews 110
Iyengar, B.K.S. 11

Jacobson, Edmund 9

Knees 49 – 50

Laryngitis 17
Lifting 32, 86, 112
Light On Yoga 11
Lloyd, Amber 11
Lumbago 17, 86 – 87

Migraine 11, 87 – 90
Mitchell, Laura 9

Neck 22, 31, 43 – 44, 105, 109, 119
Nervous breakdown 90 – 91
Nervousness 113
Nursing 111 – 113

Once A Month 95
Overeating *see also* Anorexia 13, 78 – 79

Pain 13, 91 – 93
Painkillers 20, 91
Panic 11, 93 – 95, 108
Pelvis 48 – 49
Performing 113
Phobias 11, 75 – 76
Pins and needles 22, 105
Pregnancy 114

Pre-menstrual tension 95 – 96

Reading 33, 79
Relaxation For Living 11

Self-help For Your Nerves 76
Shock 16
Shoulders 22, 29 – 30, 40 – 43, 54 – 55, 105, 119
Sitting 29 – 31, 33 – 35, 86
Sleep 36, 83 – 85, 111 – 112
Smoking 13
Spine 17, 22 – 23, 109
Sport 36, 114 – 115
Standing 86
Stroke 97 – 99

T'ai Chi 96
Tension 13, 18, 28
Terminal illness 82 – 83
Thrombosis 20, 97 – 99
Tinnitus 99 – 100
Tongue 22, 45
Tranquillisers 20, 101 – 102

Ulcers 11, 17, 96 – 97

Waiting 115 – 117
Walking 25 – 28, 86, 114, 118
Watching television 33, 36, 79
Weekes, Claire 76
Work 117 – 120
Worry 11
Wrists 39

Yoga 10 – 11, 78, 82, 96, 101 – 102, 117
Yoga – 28-day Exercise Plan 11